EAT THE EIGHT:

PREVENTING FOOD ALLERGY WITH FOOD AND THE IMPERFECT ART OF MEDICINE

EAT THE EIGHT:

PREVENTING FOOD ALLERGY WITH FOOD AND THE IMPERFECT ART OF MEDICINE

RON SUNOG, MD

The Nasiona

San Francisco

Eat The Eight : Preventing Food Allergy with Food and the Imperfect Art of Medicine

Copyright © Ron Sunog, MD, 2019

Published by *The Nasiona*

For information contact :

nasiona.mail.@gmail.com

https://thenasiona.com/

Author photograph by Max Sunog

ISBN: 978-1-950124-02-2

Dedication

SOME MONTHS AFTER THE LEARNING Early About Peanut (LEAP) study was published, I attended a talk for parents about food allergy given by a prominent local pediatric allergist. Having observed little enthusiasm in the medical community for introducing peanut to infants, I wondered what a local expert was telling parents. When the speaker explained that LEAP provided strong evidence for the early introduction of peanut to infants, the mother of a teenager with peanut allergy began to cry softly. The speaker explained that this information, unfortunately, had not been known when her child was an infant. When I introduced myself as a physician and added that despite the new information little had changed in the way of physician guidance, the allergist said that his experience was much the same. The weeping mother and the other parents in attendance simply could not understand how this was so.

I dedicate this book to parents and children who have had to contend with food allergy, with the hope that fewer families will have to do so in the future.

Contents

Acknowledgments

I AM A PEDIATRICIAN IN private practice for over 30 years. What I am not is a researcher, healthy food entrepreneur, or trailblazer of any kind. But LEAP and similar studies somehow turned me into an Eat The Eight crusader; thinking and talking endlessly about food allergy, evidence based medicine, and the psychology of changing minds for the last three-and-a-half years.

First, I must thank my wife, Melissa, daughter, Emma, and son Max, for indulging me so kindly that I believe they, too, are enthralled by these topics. Their editing help was also indispensable.

Thank you Scot, Bob, and Larry, for your interest in this project and working with me on my early peanut puff ventures.

Thank you Rich, Greg, Guru Hari, Jack, and Holly, for making Puffworks baby a reality.

Thank you Steven, Jennifer, Mordie, Amy, Woody, Nancy, and Deborah; friends whose interest in peanut butter puffs and *Eat The Eight* was just so nice to have.

Thank you Sue, for reading a first draft and somehow providing helpful advice on what in retrospect was nothing but a jumble of words.

Thank you Steve—an old friend, classmate, and a pediatric

allergist—for providing the initial editing that served as a template in my mind for all my subsequent writing. Thank you Scot, Aunt Vicki, Amy, and Mordie, for your input after reading the manuscript at various stages.

Thank you Julián, my editor and publisher, for making Eat The Eight a book, but mostly for believing in this project.

And thanks, again, Melissa, because you deserve more thanks.

An Ounce of Prevention is Worth a Pound of Cure

"The whole world is a potential danger for him:

Playgrounds where another child may have left food

residue on the monkey bars. Parks where squirrel-lovers

have left behind peanut shells."

(A parent whose child is allergic to peanuts,

Commonwealth, WBUR.org, 2/27/15.)

EPIPHANY: "A MOMENT OF SUDDEN revelation or insight." I learned the meaning of this word in 10th grade English class, reading James Joyce. My high school friends and I joked that every mundane thought we had was an epiphany. On April 4, 2015, I had an epiphany.

At this point in my story I would be happy to recreate that moment—the early signs of spring, the music that was playing, the feel of the breeze—but I can't, because all that I remember is the spark of a thought in my head and then telling my wife and kids, "I just had a great idea. I'm going to develop the best, first peanut food for infants."

My idea was inspired by the remarkable results of the Learning Early About Peanut (LEAP) study that the *New England Journal of Medicine* published just two months earlier. The LEAP investigators, motivated to do the study by the fact that the prevalence of peanut allergy had been rising for years, showed decisively that *feeding a peanut food to high-risk infants significantly reduced their risk of developing peanut allergy*. This finding was widely acclaimed as a major breakthrough that would result in far-reaching changes to infant feeding practices, because the vast majority of parents withheld the "Big Eight" foods from infants— peanut, milk, shellfish, tree nut, egg, fish, and wheat, which are responsible for 90% of food allergy reactions. Parents generally believed that delaying introduction of these foods until at least one year of age decreased infants' risk of developing allergy because that is what doctors advised. Over the past decade, there were studies that looked at the possible benefit from the early introduction of other "Big Eight" foods. Although none of these studies yielded the conclusive results that LEAP had, there was some evidence that the benefits of early introduction were not limited to only peanut.

As a pediatrician for over thirty years and the father of two children, I know how important it is to all parents to keep our children safe. For the 8% of children with food allergy, including the 2.5% who have peanut allergy, the everyday experience of being around food, the necessary and usually joyful act of eating, can pose a danger. As you might expect, the parents of these children experience significant anxiety and stress.

I anticipated with enthusiasm the feeding guidelines that I believed would be quickly forthcoming from the National Institute of Health (NIH) and the American Academy of Pediatrics (AAP), the institutions that doctors would look to for specific recommendations about what to advise parents based on the LEAP study. And I knew parents would need guidance regarding exactly how to introduce peanut to their infants, because infants cannot eat peanuts or undiluted peanut butter due to the risk of choking.

The NIH, however, did not announce new infant feeding guidelines for almost a year after the publication of LEAP, and they seemed too narrowly focused. Only a small minority of doctors began to advise parents about the early introduction of peanut to infants. Further, parents I spoke with, both in my office and during conversations in my pursuit of the perfect first peanut food for infants, were dubious and apprehensive.

I had reasoned that with food allergy so common, and the anxiety it can provoke so unsettling, if we had a treatment that could decrease a child's risk of developing food allergy, every pediatrician would be talking about it and every parent would be interested. If this treatment were not only extraordinarily safe but also had additional health benefits, every parent would enthusiastically embrace it. Now we had something that was all this and more, because it would *prevent* a problem rather than treat it after it occurred; because it was not a medication, a vaccine, or a procedure, so there would be no co-pays, or side effects, or additional visits to the doctor; because this incredible new "treatment" was nothing more than healthful foods.

Yet, it was abundantly evident that the results of LEAP and other infant feeding studies did not have the impact on institutions, doctors, and parents that I had envisioned.

Eat The Eight explores why. The process of searching for the best first peanut food for infants took me on an unexpected, sometimes circuitous, and ultimately enlightening route; from the outdated feeding advice and the origins of our food allergy epidemic, to the methodology behind expert recommendations and medical advice, to the psychology that underpins the way we accept or reject new facts.

Much of what I discovered was surprising and even a bit disconcerting, but confirmed for me that preventing food allergy with food makes enormous sense despite the obstacles to this simple solution. It is my hope that *Eat The Eight* will provide some insight into the art of medicine and that you will agree.

CHAPTER I

The Prevalence and Burden of Food Allergy

"The only thing that scares me more than needing the

Epi-pen is not having the Epi-pen when I need it."

(Tiffany Glass Ferreira, foodallergyfun.com)

WITH AN ESTIMATED 4% OF adults allergic to some food, we live in a society where we regularly encounter concern about food allergy. The current situation is sometimes described as an epidemic. The parents of children with food allergy may be anxious, of course, but we are all made conscious of food allergy whenever we read a menu that reminds us to "let your server know if you have a food allergy," when the airline attendant announces that someone on board has severe peanut allergy and no peanut snacks should be opened, when we can't send our children to school with a peanut butter sandwich.

Although precise statistics are difficult to obtain, a Centers for Disease Control and Prevention study done in 2013 showed that food allergies among children increased approximately 50% between 1997 and 2011 and today approximately 8% of children have an allergy to one or more foods. To put this in perspective: the average classroom has two children with food allergy; of the 4,000,000 infants born this year, we can expect 320,000 to develop an allergy to some food.

The Big Eight are responsible for 90% of food allergy reactions. Among children with food allergy:

—25.2% are allergic to peanut

—21.1% to milk

—17.2% to shellfish

—13.1% to tree nut

—9.8% to egg

—6.2% to fish

—5% to wheat

—4.6% to soy

About 30% of children with food allergy are allergic to more than one food. Although some allergies can be outgrown, allergies to peanut, tree nuts, fish, and shellfish are usually life-long.

Food allergy exacts a significant health toll. Reactions can occur within seconds or minutes of exposure to the offending food, but sometimes even hours later; are unpredictable; and can include hives, itching, facial swelling, vomiting, anxiety, difficulty breathing, a drop in blood pressure, and loss of consciousness. These symptoms can occur singly or in combination.

When allergy symptoms occur in combination involving more than one organ system, it is called anaphylaxis. Anaphylaxis can occur with allergic reaction to any substance and is sometimes life threatening. Outside of the hospital (where medications are the most common cause), food is the most common cause.

When anaphylaxis is severe it can cause death within minutes, generally from asphyxiation caused by swelling in the throat or from a severe drop in blood pressure and collapse of the cardiovascular system. Although it can also be mild and resolve on its own, the unpredictable nature of its course dictates that every case be treated as a life-threatening emergency, requiring epinephrine and often other medications. Along with the increasing numbers of children with food allergy, there has been an enormous increase in the number of cases of anaphylaxis. In 2016, the *Journal of Allergy and Clinical Immunology* reported that "from 2005 through 2014 children from 5 to 7 years of age had an increase of 285% in food-related anaphylaxis and children from 0 to 4 years had a 479% increase." After treatment in an emergency room, a patient must be observed for hours, as symptoms can return even after they have responded to treatment and resolved.

Needless to say, anaphylaxis can be terrifying, for both the patient and observers. I experienced this in my own living room when a cousin failed to mention his peanut allergy and then ate a forkful of my wife's homemade coleslaw with Asian peanut dressing. He quickly turned red, developed hives on his face and arms, and soon had difficulty breathing. He reached for his Epi-Pen (epinephrine auto-injector for emergency treatment) only to discover he had left it at home. Fortunately, with an emergency room very close by, he was treated and recovered quickly. It is important to note that although death from anaphylaxis is rare, not having access to epinephrine increases that risk. *Everyone with food allergy should have an epinephrine auto-injector available at all times.* (On a more recent visit, my cousin proudly displayed the Epi-Pen he now dutifully carries at all times.)

According to Food Allergy Research and Education (FARE), a preeminent non-profit organization:

—"Every three minutes, a food allergy reaction sends someone to the emergency room.

—Each year in the U.S., 200,000 people require emergency medical care for allergic reactions to food.

—Childhood hospitalizations for food allergy tripled between the late 1990s and the mid-2000s.

—About 40 percent of children with food allergies have experienced a severe allergic reaction such as anaphylaxis."

The annual number of U.S. deaths attributable to food allergy is difficult to ascertain, but has been estimated in various studies to range between about 10 and 200. Since these figures are derived from hospital diagnoses and death certificates, it is exceedingly difficult to be accurate. A hospital visit or death from food allergy reaction may be recorded as being the result of its proximate cause, cardiovascular collapse or asthma for example, rather than anaphylaxis.

In addition to the health cost, the financial cost to society from food allergy is estimated at about $25 billion a year, which includes expenses for medical intervention, medications, and dietary interventions. The additional average annual expense of raising a child with food allergy is over $4,000.

Having food allergy also predisposes one to other problems, resulting in a ripple effect in terms of burden to individual and society. Some patients experience what allergists refer to as the "atopic or allergic march," a progression of allergic diseases that often begin early in life with eczema (also referred to as atopic dermatitis) and proceeds to food allergy, hay fever (also referred to as allergic rhinitis), and, finally, asthma. Compared to children without food allergy, those with food allergy are 2-4 times more likely to have related conditions such as asthma and other allergies. Recent research has shown that children with eczema who develop food allergy are seven times as likely to develop asthma as children with eczema who have not developed food allergy.

A lot of the anxiety around food allergy results from how difficult it can be to avoid exposure. Most children who require medical treatment for a reaction at school were known to have an allergy prior to the reaction. Put another way, even when children and their teachers know they have food allergy and are aware of the need for caution, accidental exposures and reactions occur frequently. It has been reported that over 15 percent of school-aged children with food allergies have had a reaction in school.

Beyond the obvious concern about anaphylaxis, food allergic children and their families also experience emotional distress because of social and other implications. A psychology professor friend of mine has described the isolation of the school lunch table for the kids with food allergy as "a social Siberia," and about one-third of children with food allergy have been bullied as a result. A survey of parents of children with food allergy revealed that they, too, experience significant emotional impact. Families of peanut allergic children are more fearful about diet and health impacts than even the families of children with diabetes.

The passage of a law in Canada in 2006 designed to protect children with food allergy had unintended consequences that shed light on the emotional issues these children sometimes have. After the tragic death of a 13-year-old student from anaphylaxis in a school in Ontario in 2003, policies were enacted to accommodate and protect students who had food allergy. Schools were required to reduce students' exposure to allergens and to train teachers to manage allergic reactions. As a result, children with food allergy became much more visible in schools. A study published in 2016 found that along with the benefits of greater awareness of food allergy and allergic reactions, these children felt stigmatized and excluded. As one child interviewed for the study put it, when others become aware of your food allergy, "Automatically, you are tagged as a person who is different...you are on the outside."

It is fairly plain to see that an intervention that could result in fewer children with food allergy would be of enormous benefit to the child, their family, and society.

CHAPTER II

Guidelines Without Evidence

"Extraordinary claims require extraordinary evidence."

(Carl Sagan)

THE FOOD ALLERGY EPIDEMIC ENCOMPASSES many foods. For example, findings presented at the American College of Allergy, Asthma, and Immunology (ACAAI) annual meeting in October 2017 noted that allergy to cashews is on the rise. Also, an analysis of physician billing data in August 2017 showed that from 2007 to 2016 the diagnosis of food allergy in general increased by 70% in urban areas and 110% in rural areas. The proliferation of allergy diagnoses along with increased media coverage and a heightened awareness by the public has left us with many questions. Although not limited to peanut, a good way to gain insight into the broad food allergy epidemic is to look at the history of allergy to peanut.

Accounts of food allergy date at least as far back as Hippocrates's writings from around 400 BCE and there are known case reports of reactions to food in the medical literature from the

1600s, but one review suggested that they may date back to dietary advice for pregnant women and individuals with skin lesions from Chinese Emperors around 2735 BCE. Although peanut allergy, specifically, has no doubt existed for a very long time, up until the late 1980's the only known recorded case of death from anaphylactic reaction to peanut was in 1982. In 1988, there were four such deaths reported in the US and one in Canada. There were four more reported in the US between 1989 and 1992. In May of 1990, the *British Medical Journal* (BMJ) published a report of four cases of fatal anaphylaxis: a 23-year-old man who had eaten a meal of Chinese food that included satay sauce, which is made with peanuts; a 20-year-old man who had eaten a meal that he did not know contained nuts; a 21-year-old man who had eaten a "dried food dressing" made with nuts; and a 15-year-old boy who had eaten a piece of cake made with nuts. All four had known they were allergic to peanut and avoided foods they knew to have peanut; all four reacted to food they believed to be free of peanut; and all four died despite intensive medical intervention. The report noted, "All four were aware of their allergies *but could not avoid the allergen*" (italics mine). In that same volume of the *BMJ*, there appeared the report of a 28-year-old woman who had believed she was eating a beef hamburger, but was instead eating a "vegetableburger" made with peanuts. It was titled "Vegetableburger Allergy: All Was Nut as It Appeared" and made note of "the potential danger of vegetarian food to the beef burger eating, peanut allergic, carnivore..." Deputy Editor of the Journal, Dr. Tony Smith, wrote an editorial emphasizing that peanut may turn up unexpectedly in small amounts in a variety of foods, unlike, for example, oysters or strawberries, and that even the cautious person with peanut allergy is at risk. A letter to the editor in

June highlighted the risk of inadvertent exposure, noting that peanut oil can be an unexpected component of some foods. A letter to the editor the following month called the case reports "depressing reading." As a result of these reports, by the early 1990s, the medical community took far more notice of peanut allergy. It is now clear that this increase in the number of reports did not mean there was necessarily an increase in the number of cases, because (as noted in the last chapter) deaths due to peanut anaphylaxis were sometimes given a different diagnosis in the hospital or recorded differently on the death certificate. Nevertheless, in 1992, *Pediatric Annals* stated that the most worrisome food allergy problem for pediatricians was peanut allergy, because peanut appeared to be the most dangerous of the allergenic foods. Besides the number of case reports, it seems quite likely that a lot of the worry was driven by their implication that for even the careful peanut allergic individual, a potentially life-threatening anaphylactic reaction was unavoidable and possibly untreatable.

The public grew increasingly concerned about peanut allergy and the pressure on medical researchers to find a remedy grew in tandem. Unfortunately, there were no robust studies on which to base interventions that might prevent people from developing food allergies. In the absence of good evidence, they would have done well to follow the dictum, "Don't just do something, stand there"—but that's not what occurred.

In 1989, the *Journal of Allergy and Clinical Immunology* stated that, "*reduced exposure* of infants to allergenic foods appeared to reduce food sensitization and allergy" (italics mine) despite the lack of any compelling evidence to support this assertion. A study done in 1995 compared infants who followed standard feeding practices—no restrictions on eating potentially allergenic foods—to infants who were not fed these foods and whose mothers also avoided these foods. These infants were not fed cow's milk until age one year, egg until age two years, and peanut and fish until age three years. Their mothers avoided those same foods during the last trimester of pregnancy and while breast feeding. Although the avoidance group did have a lower prevalence of food allergy before age two years, by three years the groups had no difference in milk allergy, and by seven years they had no difference in food allergy, eczema, asthma, or allergic rhinitis. Delayed introduction may have delayed, but did not prevent, the development of food allergy.

Practicing physicians were as anxious to offer parents a way to reduce their infants' risk of developing food allergy as researchers had been to provide guidance. Despite the lack of supporting evidence, they began to preach delayed introduction of the Big Eight foods to infants, and by the late 1990s this advice had become gospel. In August of 2000, the AAP Committee on Nutrition established infant feeding guidelines which it described as reasonable, although it was acknowledged that there were no conclusive studies on which to base definitive recommendations. It stated that, "Solid foods should not be introduced into the diet of high-risk infants until 6 months of age, with dairy products delayed until 1 year, eggs until 2 years, and peanuts, nuts, and fish until 3 years of age." The practice of delaying the introduction of certain foods to infants became widespread and the prevalence of food allergies soared, peanut allergy dramatically so. What had seemed like reasonable recommendations might not have been so reasonable after all.

How could the AAP make infant feeding recommendations without good evidence to support them? As it turns out, until the relatively recent past a great deal of medical advice was dispensed without the support of good evidence. The very term "evidence-based medicine" (EBM) is relatively new.

Some credit Dr. Gordon Guyatt of McMaster University in Ontario with introducing the term in the 1990's, defining it as an approach to clinical decision-making based on the analysis of published research. Colleagues did not embrace Guyatt's use of the term. Although they acknowledged clinical decisions were often made without a firm scientific foundation, they were offended by the obvious implications. I myself recall being quite surprised when I began to hear the term used early in my career—hadn't everything I had learned been based on evidence?

A review published in 2004 noted that although people were increasingly interested in being shown persuasive evidence as the basis for making informed choices about health care, good evidence that could be applied broadly to many patients in various settings was not readily available. It was suggested that possibly as few as one-third of medical services were supported by compelling evidence that the benefit was greater than the harm.

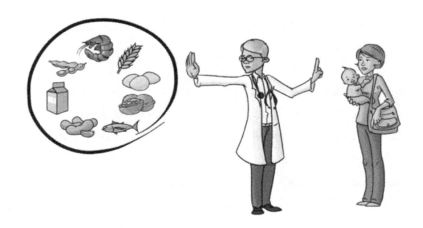

AAP Guidelines, August 2000

Utilizing EBM, the doctor patient relationship ought to become less hierarchical and more collaborative. A doctor would no longer simply recommend, "you should do this" or "you shouldn't do that." Instead, the aggregate of evidence for a recommendation would be carefully evaluated for its quality, quantity, and consistency and then given a rating. Several such rating scales exist including one, for example, that classifies recommendations as A-level when based on evidence determined to be consistent and of high quality; B-level when based on evidence determined to be inconsistent or of limited-quality; and C-level when based on consensus, usual practice, and opinion.

In practice, a physician would present to the patient what is believed to be true, the strength of the evidence for this belief, and a recommendation based on this. Our approach to treating ear infections and how we present that to parents is a prime example of one way EBM has changed pediatrics. At a recent office visit, upon diagnosing an ear infection in a somewhat distressed and uncomfortable but not very ill-appearing six-year-old Devin, I informed his mother that it is well-established that many ear infections are caused by a virus and will resolve without antibiotics, so not prescribing antibiotics is a reasonable option in many instances. Avoiding an unnecessary course of antibiotics has the advantages of avoiding a possible allergic reaction, for which the risk is low; a mild side effect, for which the risk is moderate; and saves the expense of the medication. If Devin did not improve in 24-48 hours I could prescribe an antibiotic at that point. Foregoing treatment at this time carried the small risk that Devin would have an uncomfortable day or two that might have been improved by antibiotics and might require a follow up visit that might otherwise not have been necessary. An untreated bacterial ear infection can lead to complications, but if Devin did not improve and his mother brought him back, the risk of this would be extremely small. During the early years of my career, when upon examining a child I detected an ear infection, I would simply inform the parent of the diagnosis and prescribe an antibiotic. Devin's mother, who was concerned about the overuse of antibiotics, felt confident that she could make Devin comfortable with ibuprofen and calculated that this approach would likely be successful. She elected to observe Devin at home and follow up as needed.

The utility of EBM is evident, but it places significant responsibility on practicing physicians and patients. Are physicians adequately trained and prepared to analyze the studies and weigh the data? In other words, are doctors able to determine which studies yield strong evidence and which do not and then apply their assessment appropriately? Can patients properly consider the strength of evidence when weighing their options?

Canadian physician and author Dr. Kevin Patterson described in 2002 the entrenched chain of command that has long existed in the medical profession, with the experts and researchers directing the specialists, who in turn direct the generalists, who then direct the patients. More recent studies indicate that this has not changed. In 2012, a paper by British physician and Professor of Public Health, Dr. John Gabbay, explored how most doctors acquire information, noting they rarely read, evaluate, or directly use evidence from research. Instead, they are informed somewhat by brief reading, but mostly by their interactions with each other, opinion leaders, and other sources, including pharmaceutical company reps. Given its complexity, it should come as no surprise that doctors generally eschew the original research. Dr. Kevin Barraclough of the University of Bristol Medical School commented in the *BMJ*, "Of all the areas of math, probability and [...] statistics are the most slippery to grasp [...] doctors, including myself, don't understand it." He opined that such data inserted into research papers with the supposed intent of illuminating information served instead to obscure it. (Another clinician responded that this was so because the papers were written to be published rather than to be read.)

Unfortunately, the very same experts that practicing physicians rely on to evaluate the studies might also have difficulty determining which studies provide strong evidence for their findings. In the *New Atlantis Journal of Technology and Society,* Ivan Oransky, global editorial director of *MedPage Today* wondered "Why should we expect that a few experts, *who may not really be experts at all in the techniques used in a given study* (italics mine), would be able to spot every error?" And if expert reviewers making a good faith effort to review research papers cannot always spot data that doesn't support the researchers' conclusions, it follows as no surprise that even journals that adhere to very careful review standards publish papers that should be and sometimes are retracted. Further, despite the fact that many published papers are retracted annually, it's possible that many more ought to be. Richard Smith, a former editor of the *BMJ*, claimed in 1988 "only 5% of published papers reached minimum standards of scientific soundness and clinical relevance, and in most journals the figure was less than 1%." A 2017 editorial in *Journal Anaesthesia* wondered if "the flood of retractions is about to become a tsunami." It simply is not to be expected that the average—or even the unusually skilled—doctor will easily or always recognize flawed research.

To be fair, the way doctors acquire information is completely consistent with how we all do. As author Elizabeth Kolbert so eloquently put it, "We've been relying on one another's expertise ever since we figured out how to hunt together [...] So well do we collaborate[...] that we can hardly tell where our own understanding ends and others' begins." Unsurprisingly, when it comes to the options for treating ear infections, my knowledge and the knowledge of my peers comes from reading review articles written by the experts, attending conferences where experts present information, and discussions we have with each other—not from analyzing the original research that has led to the recommendations.

In my experience, day-to-day practice remains largely unchanged despite the advent of EBM—the clinician often defers to the expert academicians and researchers, while patients generally defer to their health care provider. These recommendations may now come with qualifiers regarding the strength of the underlying evidence, but those very qualifiers are presented by the experts. Physicians and patients alike make the general assumption that the recommendations *must be backed by credible evidence*—why else would they have been made?

Though parents do increasingly seek credible evidence, that evidence can be difficult to process. For example, although after more than thirty years in practice I am well versed in the risks and benefits of vaccines, understanding the complexity of those risks and benefits can be daunting for parents. It is true that having that discussion with a parent in my office sometimes does enable them to make what for some is a difficult decision. At the same time, if they are uncertain or hesitant, often what they really want to know is "Did you give this vaccine to your children?" For those parents, the answer to that question provides them with a proxy about the safety and efficacy of the vaccine rather than having to contemplate the minutiae of rare but potentially significant side effects.

Many parents have already made up their mind about vaccines before I have presented any information. Those who choose to vaccinate their children seem to do so based on a general trust of the medical network—the researchers who studied the disease, the drug company that developed the vaccine, the Food and Drug Administration that approved the vaccine, their personal doctor who is recommending it, and the nurse who is administering it—that acts in coordinated fashion to provide the vaccine. Those who decline the vaccine seem more influenced by reports of side effects (sometimes anecdotal and unsubstantiated, but broadly disseminated on the internet), the untrustworthy behavior of big pharma, and a belief in the protection provided by nature, healthy living, or god. Again, these decisions are based not so much on an accounting of the presented risks and benefits, but rather on trust in whichever experts parents have chosen to defer to.

This is not to disparage the importance or potential benefits of EBM or to suggest that it has made no difference at all. After all, 20 years ago Devin would have simply received an antibiotic for his ear infection. Presenting the evidence to his mother gave her the opportunity to make a different choice, which turned out to be the best course of action.

Perhaps if EBM had already advanced beyond its nascency in 2000, the AAP Committee on Nutrition would have published no new feeding guidelines at all and parents would never have been advised to delay the introduction of the Big Eight to infants. Had the AAP presented guidelines suggesting that parents delay the introduction of the Big Eight foods to infants and emphasized the caveat that the evidence for this was weak, perhaps pediatricians would have been circumspect and parents would have rejected them. And one could rightly ask what exactly was so compelling about this advice that virtually all parents would so completely adopt this particular expert recommendation over grandma's exhortation that "my generation fed all the babies those foods and no one had a problem!" As it was, the recommendation to delay the introduction of the Big Eight foods to infants was described as reasonable and treated by experts, practicing physicians, and parents alike as authoritative. Delaying the introduction of these foods became the standard, and the prevalence of food allergies, which increased by an astonishing 50% between 1997 and 2011, continues to increase to this day. Today, many parents, including the vast majority of new parents I see, still "know" with certainty that the Big Eight foods, especially anything containing peanut, should not be fed to infants until they are at least one year old. The problem with this "fact" is that this advice was dubious from the start and, as you will see, has been understood to be flat out wrong since 2008.

CHAPTER III

Can Facts Replace Folklore?

"There was a lot of folklore built around this idea that something the mother eats during pregnancy or lactation or something she feeds her baby has long-term impact for allergy disease. Traditionally a lot of pediatricians have recommended not to give infants eggs, fish, peanuts, or any nuts in the first year of life...It makes absolutely no difference."

(Dr. Frank Greer, chairperson of the AAP's Committee on Nutrition and lead author of The American Academy of Pediatrics (AAP) updated policy statement on nutritional options during pregnancy, lactation, and the first year of life, published January 2008.)

AS THE NUMBER OF CHILDREN with food allergy grew, by the mid-2000's the efficacy of delayed introduction of the Big Eight foods was being questioned. There was no evidence that withholding these foods was the actual cause of the growing prevalence of food allergy, but with time it became increasingly certain that this strategy had failed to prevent food allergy.

In January of 2008 an AAP Clinical Report acknowledged that there was no support for restricting the diet of infants beyond four to six months of age (up to which point they should take only breast milk or formula) as a way to protect against the development of allergic disease such as eczema, asthma, or food allergy. This policy statement was recognized as a major change from the recommendations put forward by the AAP in 2000, and was noted to be evidence based, in distinct contrast to the old recommendations.

To be clear, the policy did not recommend that infants should Eat The Eight, only that delaying these foods until one year of age was of no benefit. In an interview in April of 2008, Dr. Frank Greer, the lead author of the Policy Statement, stated that for children at risk for allergic disease, delaying the introduction of foods might delay the onset of allergy, but doesn't prevent allergy. (He went even further—and, we now know, too far—stating that feeding a six-month-old peanut butter has no effect at all on developing peanut allergy.)

Dr. Greer also noted that this was the strongest statement the Committee on Nutrition had published in eight years. Having garnered enormous interest from the press and from allergy groups, he was confident that the message was getting out there, yet remained concerned that pediatricians were not picking up on it.

I have been practicing pediatrics for over 30 years and believe that Dr. Greer's concerns were valid. In my experience it remained common practice to persist in the recommendation to delay the introduction of these foods or to not recommend specifically that there was no benefit to delaying them. A study of Canadian physicians published only five months ago found that some continue to recommend delayed introduction of allergenic foods. I am not aware of a similar study of US physicians, but I suspect the same is true.

That the new policy was not quickly and widely adopted may have been unfortunate but is, perhaps, understandable. We live in an age of information overload. It was estimated in 2009 that we can be subject to as many as 100,000 words and 34 GB (there are thousands of pages in every GB of data) of information daily. In 2012, the paper "Doctors and Medical Science" noted that 1.29 peer-reviewed papers are published every minute. It goes without saying that physicians are subject to incredible volumes of new and important information that competes for our attention and none of us can keep up with all of it. Regrettably, pediatricians seemed to take less notice of this particular Policy Statement than some had hoped.

I happened to be particularly attuned to this information in 2008 for a simple reason: having been an overweight child, by the time I was a teenager I had become very interested in nutrition and I have maintained this interest throughout my career.

My experience also supports the notion that parents' attitudes about this were—and continue to be—difficult to change. As Mark Twain is purported to have said, *"It ain't what you don't know that gets you into trouble. It's what you know for sure that just ain't so."* And despite the new information, most parents knew for sure that infants should not eat the Big Eight foods, although this just wasn't so.

It is now widely understood that entrenched beliefs can be extraordinarily difficult to let go of and new evidence often does not help change minds. This somehow still feels astonishing, although it should no longer be surprising, since psychology research has validated this concept since the 1970's. In February 2017, Elizabeth Kolbert wrote in *The New Yorker*, "Everyone who's followed the research—or even occasionally picked up a copy of *Psychology Today*—knows, any graduate student with a clipboard can demonstrate that reasonable-seeming people are often totally irrational." Researchers have concluded that people often fail to revise their beliefs, even after evidence for those beliefs has been completely discredited. I prove this concept to myself daily as my own mind clings to the idea that facts *must* be able to change minds, despite strong evidence to the contrary. This phenomenon is known as confirmation bias, the "tendency people have to embrace information that supports their beliefs and reject information that contradicts them."

In addition to confirmation bias, there can be little doubt that new information perceived to be untrustworthy is unlikely to change minds. Although it is the very nature of science that conclusions change as more is learned, new recommendations can lead to skepticism about the reliability of experts and the advice they dispense. There is perhaps nowhere this is more manifest than in the field of nutrition. While this can be explained by the relative newness of nutrition research, the difficulty of designing good nutrition studies, and the incorrect interpretation and sensationalization of the research in the general media, one can hardly be surprised if the public is sometimes suspicious of or difficult to convince with new facts. In an article published in *The Journal of the American Medical Association* (JAMA) in August 2018, Dr. John Ioannidis, Professor of Medicine and of Health Research and Policy at Stanford University School of Medicine and a Professor of Statistics at Stanford University School of Humanities and Sciences, went so far as to suggest that the entire field of nutritional research is in need of basic reform because it has become so disconnected from sound scientific principles.

Possible malfeasance on the part of researchers can also make the public wary of new findings and, therefore, less likely to adopt them. As expressed eloquently in the journal *Anesthesiology*, "The responsible conduct of research is the bedrock on which the scientific enterprise rests. *Scientific integrity is indispensable for preserving the public trust* (italics mine) and the trust of the scientific community[...] Research misconduct has become an all too familiar stain on the research and clinical landscape, and it is occurring with increasing frequency and public awareness." While the number of published research papers increased by 40% between 2000 and 2010, the number of papers retracted during that period increased by 900%. Fully two-thirds of the retractions were due to research misconduct (the rest being due to honest errors).

Regrettably, one need look no further than the recent press to find noteworthy incidents of tainted research. On June 15, 2018, Dr. Francis Collins, Director of the NIH, shut down a study of the effect of alcohol on health because the lead investigator, Dr. Kenneth Mukamal, and some of the NIH's own staff had committed egregious ethical abuses. Alcoholic beverage company executives had pledged $66 million of the $100 million in funding to conduct a 10-year-long randomized trial, the results of which they had hoped to use for promotional purposes. Dr. Mukamal, a Harvard scientist, had conferred in secret with these executives and carefully designed the trial to study the possible cardiac benefits of having one drink a day while making it very difficult to detect possible harms from drinking. He reassured the executives that even if no benefit were proven, no harm would be shown, so the results would counter the World Health Organization pronouncement that any consumption of alcohol carries risk.

In September 2018, it was revealed that Dr. José Baselga, the chief medical officer at Memorial Sloan Kettering Cancer Center in New York, failed to disclose millions of dollars in payments he had received from drug and health care companies that were related to research he had done. While there has not been any proof of biased research, the concern for this is inescapable.

Some experts contend that the increased retractions are a measure that the system is working and that this should reassure the public. It is also true that despite the enormous increase in the number of retracted papers, the total number represents just 1 out of 2000 published studies. On the other hand, despite the proverb (immortalized by the Osmonds and the Jackson 5) "one bad apple don't spoil the whole bunch," the whole bunch may be thought of as spoiled by a doubting public. Exploring the psychology behind holding a corporation responsible for the acts of individuals, a law journal study concluded it is the appearance that the individuals are part of a tightly unified whole that leads to judgments of collective responsibility. It seems the public sometimes applies that same psychology to medical facts and advice, treating all medical researchers and research institutions as a monolith and holding them collectively guilty for the sins of a few. (For the record, one bad apple can literally spoil the whole bunch.)

A prime example of how facts can be impotent is observed in multiple controversies implicating vaccines as the cause of autism, which originated with the publication of a study in the *Lancet*, a prestigious British medical journal, in 1998. Dr. Andrew Wakefield and his associates described a group of twelve children who exhibited symptoms of autism and also evidence of measles virus present in their digestive tract after having received the MMR (measles, mumps, German measles) vaccine. Although no causal relationship had been shown between the vaccine and autism, Wakefield released a video that suggested otherwise, claiming that autism was the result of the combination vaccine. He then recommended administration of each component of the vaccine separately, on different days, rather than all at once in combination. Parents became frightened of the MMR vaccine and many declined or delayed its administration to their children.

Over the next 12 years, many well-designed studies showed no link between **MMR** and autism, but the damage had been done. The new extremely well-supported facts did not change minds; many parents in Britain deferred or declined the **MMR** vaccine, and the number of children who contracted measles increased.

Years later, it was discovered that Wakefield had conflicts of interest, having been paid by attorneys seeking to sue the vaccine manufacturers and having filed for a patent for a single component measles vaccine in 1997. The *Lancet* retracted Wakefield's study; soon after, he was banned from the practice of medicine in Britain. Dr. Wakefield and his research had been discredited, but what were parents to do now? If the *Lancet*—a medical journal held in very high esteem—was to be trusted, why had it published the deeply flawed study in the first place? It was known that Dr. Wakefield might have been influenced by monetary gain. Was the same true for those with contrary views?

Additional controversies about vaccines and autism have focused on the preservative thimerosal that has been used in some vaccines. These persist despite the fact that *many large studies affording a high degree of statistical power, from several different countries, performed by a number of different researchers, and utilizing a variety of methods, have shown that autism is not caused by thimerosal or MMR vaccine.* (Thimerosal, a mercury-based preservative, was removed from all childhood vaccines except multi-dose flu vaccine vials in 2001, despite the lack of evidence that it caused harm.)

Further investigation of the controversy over vaccines illuminates just how confounding our relationship to facts can be. On the one hand, in October 2017 it was reported that the attitudes of most parents in Britain towards the **MMR** vaccine *ultimately did change* as it became accepted that Dr. Wakefield's research was false. As parents' fear of the vaccine declined over a 20-year period the rate of vaccination went up, the number of measles infections went down, and measles was proclaimed by global health experts to have been eliminated in the UK. On the other hand, although the turnaround in Britain was encouraging, it by no means indicates an end to vaccine controversies or that the public has complete confidence in facts regarding vaccines. A recent survey of Americans by the American Society for Microbiology showed that compared to ten years ago, fewer believe it is very important for parents to have their children vaccinated, fewer believe vaccines are very important to the health of our society, and fewer have confidence in experts ability to verify the safety of vaccines. At the same time, an increasing number of States are granting non-medical exemptions from required vaccines, which has led to fewer vaccinated children. As a result, measles, a disease that was essentially eliminated from the U.S. in 2000, is being seen in growing numbers of children. Perhaps this situation will change with time as it did in Britain; possibly only after the increasing prevalence of children with measles becomes a more widely realized and accepted fact.

It is abundantly clear that understanding, accepting, and acting on facts is no simple thing. My office policy to inform and educate parents, but not refuse medical care to their children if they refuse vaccines, is reflective of this. At the same time, the ability of the human mind to embrace positions that appear to be at odds with one another is impressive. We demand evidence for recommendations, yet we often disregard the evidence and defer to the recommendations of experts when considering a medical treatment. Yet despite the paradox that our incorrect beliefs can be reinforced by facts that discredit them, when presented facts for long enough, we are capable of changing our beliefs.

Despite the unequivocal basis in fact of the new feeding guidelines established by the AAP in 2008, parents and physicians alike failed to embrace them. There was no broad campaign to promote this change and there is good reason to believe that such a transformation in entrenched infant feeding habits might require an enormous effort. A particularly apt illustration of this is the "Safe to Sleep" (formerly known as "Back To Sleep") campaign, which shares fascinating parallels to the barriers encountered when trying to change infant feeding recommendations.

Infants in the US had traditionally been put to sleep on their stomach because parents "knew" that it reduced the risk of choking on spit-up and that it was the safest sleep position. This was brought into question when it was observed that in other countries infants slept safely on their back and in those same countries the rate of

Sudden Infant Death Syndrome (SIDS, also referred to as crib-death) appeared to be lower. Research then confirmed that infants who slept on their back had a significantly reduced risk of SIDS and, contrary to common belief, did not have an increased risk of choking from spit-up. (Of note, the research on peanut consumption by infants, which I will discuss in the next chapter, was similarly inspired by the observation of practices in other countries.) In 1992, the AAP recommended that babies be placed on their back or side to sleep to reduce the risk of SIDS. In 1994, The National Institute of Child Health and Human Development launched a massive and impressive "Back To Sleep" campaign, as described by the NIH at NIH.gov:

"They began mailing campaign materials to the membership of the AAP and the American College of Obstetricians and Gynecologists, all U.S. hospitals with newborn nurseries, and regional and local clinics of the Special Supplemental Nutrition Program for Women, Infants, and Children (WIC). Public service announcements (PSAs) were sent to 6,700 radio stations and 1,000 TV stations to amplify the message that placing infants on their backs to sleep can reduce the risk of SIDS."

After this enormous outreach and very substantial investment of time and money, it was reported in August 2017—a full 23 years into the campaign—that 77 percent of parents usually and 44 percent always put their babies to sleep on their back. This is evidence of progress to be sure, but clear evidence as well that change does not come easy. Consistent with this it has been my experience over the years of this effort, which has spanned most of my career, that new parents have become increasingly comfortable with and understand the importance of putting their baby to sleep on his/her back.

With the growing incidence of food allergy and the slow acceptance of the 2008 AAP Policy Statement by the medical community, in 2010 NIH researchers did their own review of the literature and published guidelines for the diagnosis and management of food allergy. These guidelines affirmed the AAP recommendation that solid foods, including potential allergens, not be restricted after four to six months of age unless an infant is actually experiencing allergic reactions to food.

In other words, *there is no reason for a parent to delay the introduction of any food* (for the purpose of preventing food allergy) beyond four to six months of age for the vast majority of infants. Yet, the NIH guidelines, like the preceding AAP policy, failed to energize the medical community. Among parents, delayed introduction continued virtually unabated. They continued to fear that feeding their infant allergenic foods too early in life would lead to an allergic reaction.

At the time that the AAP report and the NIH guidelines were being developed, the question of early introduction for *food allergy prevention* lingered. There had been some studies suggesting that early introduction of foods might in fact prevent food allergy. Dr. Greer noted that one study showed evidence that *delayed introduction* of egg until after six months *increased the likelihood* of developing egg allergy, and in Europe it was recommended that wheat be introduced between four and six months in order to reduce the likelihood of developing wheat allergy.

Despite a growing feeling that early introduction of the Big Eight foods was not only safe but possibly beneficial, caution among US experts precluded any such recommendation. More definitive recommendations for early introduction would require strong evidence. Fortunately, researchers had already begun accumulating this very evidence.

CHAPTER IV

The Shift to Early Introduction: My Search for a Peanut Food for Infants

"It's more than mumbo-jumbo, it's a mess that has to change.

It has no basis in science."

(Canadian Allergist Dr. Milton Gold, commenting on recommendations to delay the introduction of allergenic foods to infants, quoted by Gwen Smith in "Food Allergy, A LEAP into an Allergic Culture Change," 3/15/2016.)

BY 2008 IT WAS EVIDENT that delaying the introduction of the Big Eight foods did not decrease an infants' risk of developing food allergy, therefore there was no reason to delay the introduction of these foods. As the prevalence of food allergy had actually gone up concurrent with the practice of delaying these foods, there was concern that this practice had been not only unnecessary, but also possibly responsible for the increasing numbers of children with food allergy. But this may have been nothing but coincidence—association does not prove causation. To find the cause of the growing allergy problem, researchers have examined a variety of theories.

In June 2008, Dr. Gideon Lack, Head of the Children's Allergy Service at Guy's and St. Thomas' National Health Service (NHS) Foundation Trust and Professor of Pediatric Allergy at King's College London, published a review examining a number of theories about the cause of food allergy, including decreased consumption of animal fat and decreased consumption of fresh fruit and vegetables; both Vitamin D deficiency and Vitamin D excess; the theory that decreased exposure to germs causes an increase in allergic and autoimmune disease, known as the hygiene hypothesis; and the theory that most intrigued him, the possibility that food allergy is developed when an individual is exposed to food allergens through the skin, suggesting that exposure to these allergens through eating promotes tolerance (rather than allergy) to food. This final theory, known as the dual-allergen-exposure hypothesis, seemed both to fit well with a number of established facts about food allergy—such as the observation that in societies where a particular food is not consumed and therefore is not present in the environment, allergy to that food does not occur—and to support predictions about food allergy that were testable—by, for example, comparing infants who were fed allergenic foods to those who were not.

In November 2008, Dr. Lack and his associate Dr. George Du Toit, Consultant Pediatric Allergist with NHS at Guy's & St. Thomas' Hospitals, published a paper noting that despite guidelines that recommended avoidance of peanut during infancy in the US, UK, and Australia, peanut allergy had increased in these countries.

They observed in particular that peanut allergy (PA) prevalence appeared to be much lower in Israel, where infants freely ate a peanut-containing snack during infancy. Their study confirmed not only that Jewish children in the UK did in fact develop peanut allergy at ten times the rate of Jewish children in Israel, but also that it was difficult to attribute this difference to something other than the early introduction of peanut to infants (because they controlled for other factors, such as differences in social class, genetic background, and the particular variety of peanuts consumed). They concluded, "Israeli infants consume peanut in high quantities in the first year of life, whereas UK infants avoid peanuts. *These findings raise the question of whether early introduction of peanut during infancy, rather than avoidance, will prevent the development of PA.*" (italics mine)

To answer this question with great confidence would require a randomized controlled trial (RCT), the gold standard of clinical research—so that is precisely what Drs. Lack and Du Toit set out to do. LEAP enrolled infants with severe eczema and/or egg allergy—who were determined to be at higher risk for developing peanut allergy by the LEAP Screening Study—and randomized them to either consume or avoid peanut food. Subjects entered the study at four to 11 months of age and continued until five years of age. LEAP would take five years to complete and would be the first gold standard study about early introduction of allergenic foods, but previous studies had already provided some reason to believe that feeding infants the Big Eight foods might prevent food allergy:

—As far back as 2006 one study concluded that delayed initial exposure to cereal grains until after six months may increase the risk of developing wheat allergy and that delayed introduction as a guideline could not be recommended.

—In August of 2008, just seven months after the AAP established that delaying the Big Eight was of no benefit, a paper that explored the relationship between starting solids and food intolerance noted that concern about the practice of delaying foods until six months of age was increasing. The authors concluded *"Tolerance to food allergens appears to be driven by regular, early exposure to these proteins during a 'critical early window' of development."* (italics mine)

—In June 2009, Goran Wennergan, MD, PhD, from the Department of Pediatrics, University of Gothenburg, Queen Silvia Children's Hospital, Gothenburg, Sweden, wrote a paper with the provocative title "What If it is the Other Way Around? Early Introduction of Peanut and Fish Seems to Be Better Than Avoidance." Dr. Wennergan proposed that the early introduction of foods during infancy might induce tolerance, thereby preventing the development of allergy.

—In January of 2013 the inaugural issue of the *Journal of Allergy and Clinical Immunology: In Practice* did a review of the current literature and expert opinion and published recommendations for the *prevention of allergic disease* through dietary intervention, stating that new information suggests that delaying the introduction of foods to infants might increase the risk of food allergy, and *"the early introduction of allergenic foods may prevent food allergy in infants/children."* (italics mine)

—In December of 2013, the Canadian Pediatric Society in a joint statement with the Canadian Society of Allergy and Clinical Immunology stated that although research in this area was not complete, *parents should not delay the introduction of any specific foods* beyond six months of age because this would not prevent, and might even increase, the risk of developing food allergy. It was noted that the strength of evidence for this was in the middle range.

By 2014, advice to parents on authoritative pediatric blogs began to encourage early introduction. Dr. Carolyn Sax, writing for the Boston Children's Hospital health blog, noted that "[...] several studies have shown that *introduction of foods like eggs, fish, milk, and nuts during the first 12 months of life actually reduces a child's risk of developing food allergy*" (italics mine).

Dr. Todd Green, Director of the University of Pittsburgh Medical Center Allergy/Immunology Fellowship Program, wrote on the Kids with Food Allergies website "[...] there is no reason to wait until a baby is older [than four to six months] before introducing highly allergenic foods, and some *studies suggest that it may even be helpful to introduce these foods early*" (italics mine).

Again, by this time it was *fully accepted that no harm came from early introduction.* Still, an unequivocal recommendation promoting early introduction of the Big Eight would require stronger evidence.

Having commenced in 2010, LEAP was published in the venerable *New England Journal of Medicine* in February 2015. The results, universally acknowledged to be unimpeachable because the study had been so well designed and performed, demonstrated unequivocally that infants at high risk of developing peanut allergy who ate peanut early and continuously had an at least 80% lower risk of developing peanut allergy than high-risk infants for whom the introduction of peanut was intentionally delayed. LEAP had attained the Holy Grail of allergy prevention research, having shown that not only was it *not beneficial to delay the introduction* of the most notorious of the Big Eight, it was in point of fact *beneficial to introduce peanut early to high-risk infants.*

Praise for LEAP within the medical community was immediate, loud, and effusive:

—Dr. Daniel Rotrosen, Director of the Division of Allergy, Immunology, and Transplantation at the National Institute of Allergy and Infectious Disease, stated, "While recent studies showed no benefit from allergen avoidance, the LEAP study is the first to show that early introduction of dietary peanut is actually beneficial and identifies an effective approach to manage a serious public health problem." (From a National Institute of Health press release 2/23/15.)

—Anthony S. Fauci, MD, Director of The National Institute of Health and Infectious Disease, added, "For a study to show a benefit of this magnitude in the prevention of peanut allergy is without precedent. The results have the potential to transform how we approach food allergy prevention."

In addition to reaction from the medical community, the LEAP findings received prodigious coverage in the lay press throughout that year:

—February 23, in the *New York Times*, "Feeding Infants Peanut Products Could Prevent Allergies, Study Suggests."

—February 23, in *The Guardian*, "Feed Babies Peanut Products to Reverse Rise in Allergy, Say Scientists."

—February 23, in *Time*, "The Surprising Way to Treat Peanut Allergies."

—February 24, in *The Atlantic*, "Is it Really Safe to Give Infants Peanut Butter?"

—March 10, in *Slate*, "Possibly the Worst Approach—In an Effort to Protect Kids from Food Allergies, American Parents Have Been Doing the Opposite."

—July 30, in *US NEWS* and *World Report*, "Peanut Allergy Prevention: Introduce Infants Early and Often."

—October 1, in *The Washington Post*, "The New Wisdom on Nut Allergies and Infants: Pediatricians Endorse Early Exposure."

But along with the well-deserved praise, voices of caution could still be heard:

—Lynne Regent, CEO of Anaphylaxis Campaign, said: "We welcome the positive results of this important study. The research could improve the lives of those at risk of developing peanut allergy and potentially lower peanut allergy figures in the future. We look forward to seeing further developments in this area."

—Anaphylaxis Campaign Information Manager, Moira Austin, added "This is an exciting and important study that is likely to inform future guidance for parents. In the meantime, parents of atopic children should seek advice from their child's allergy specialist or treating doctor before introducing peanuts into their diet."

Despite acknowledgement as a landmark study, it appeared that the advancement from "Study Conclusions" to specific "Practice Recommendations" would require leaping over some hurdles.

To be fair, the study did have limitations:

—LEAP study children were all high-risk for peanut allergy. What, if anything, could be recommended for infants who were not high-risk?

—The medical community, still acutely aware that the previous recommendation to delay introduction of the Big Eight had turned out to be "mumbo-jumbo," was now more cognizant of the need to carefully weigh the evidence. Was the evidence strong enough?

—Despite the aforementioned reports and statements giving credence to early introduction of all the Big Eight foods, LEAP looked only at early introduction of peanut. Could we expect the NIH and AAP to say anything beyond what had already long been acknowledged—"Big Eight foods need not be withheld from infants?"

By the time I had my epiphany in April of 2015, the buzz about the LEAP study was already waning. There were as yet no official guidelines, but I remained resolute in my belief that guidelines would be forthcoming very soon, early introduction of peanut would benefit all infants, and parents would eagerly seek an infant peanut food. My years of experience as a pediatrician also give me insights into infant feeding in general. I am well aware that parents prefer baby foods that are nutritious, convenient, and inviting; the $21 billion they spend annually on baby food confirms this.

Most of the infants in the LEAP study ate Bamba, an extruded corn puff coated with peanut butter that melts enough in the mouth so that choking is not a risk. I am familiar with these puffs and I've eaten them myself, so I know they are nutritionally okay and taste good. But parents have been seeking more nutritious options for babies and I decided I would try to make or find *the best* first peanut food for infants. In addition to creating a great first peanut food, I saw this as an opportunity to provide infants with a great new food to eat when learning to feed themselves.

I began in my kitchen, where I experimented with organic brown rice and whole grain oat cereals, trying to combine them with unadulterated organic peanut butter and bake them into little O's that would be scooped up hungrily by little hands. Besides introducing peanut, I imagined they would be welcomed as a more nutritious alternative to the ubiquitous O's that are babies' most popular first finger food. When not busy experimenting with grain to peanut butter ratios, I searched for a manufacturing facility that would assume production once I got the recipe right. This proved to be an early lesson about what might be called the collateral damage of the outdated feeding guidelines and the peanut allergy epidemic. Since for many years peanut was a food that essentially no parent would feed their infant, every infant food facility I contacted had a strict no peanut policy. This disappointment was ultimately of no consequence because I had no success as a food scientist—my peanut butter O's, with gummy texture, unappealing appearance, and poor flavor, would benefit no one. The time had come to move beyond my kitchen.

I contacted several commercial kitchens in the Boston area that rented space by the hour, thinking I could do better with professional equipment. I learned that they had never rented space for making food for infants because the regulations were especially stringent. It did not take long for me to realize that I was not going to be a trailblazer in any of these kitchens, either.

Knowing that I had to go in another direction, I made the decision to find help. I would start a company and find talented, enthusiastic people with the necessary expertise to help me create a peanut food. With no experience in business or finance other than operating (with my partner) a private pediatric practice, I turned to my brother-in-law Scot, an executive at a large firm in Dallas, Texas. In possession of a sharp mind and keen intellect, he immediately recognized the benefits of a peanut food for infants. We opened a corporation and called it Arachis, Inc., named for the taxonomic classification of peanut, *Arachis hypogaea.*

The barriers to a new baby food appeared insurmountable so we decided to take a different approach. We recalled that Bamba was the peanut food eaten by most of the infants in the early introduction group in the LEAP study. On closer examination, there appeared to be much to recommend peanut butter puffs as an excellent choice. We already knew that infants could eat them without choking and could easily grasp them to feed themselves. Further, years of experience in Israel have shown that infants like peanut butter puffs.

I was also pretty familiar with other infant puffs. They were not popular when my children were little, but today they are ubiquitous. These days, when I see an infant older than six months, it's a safe bet that their diaper bag includes a canister of infant puffs. *Business Insider* noted that the global baby puff market is growing almost 7% annually and is expected to reach $1.73 billion in 2021. Despite their popularity, most infant puffs are not very nutritious.

Few are made with whole grain; many have added sugar, sometimes euphemistically described as evaporated cane juice or fruit juice concentrate to provide a thin veneer of wholesomeness; and many are barely flavored with the food that is most prominent in the name of the product, often containing less than 2% of what is ostensibly the marquee ingredient. In contrast to the typical blueberry-flavored puff that contains less than 2% blueberry, a peanut butter puff would approach or exceed a peanut butter content of 50% and would likely be the most nutritious infant puff on the shelf.

A puff begins with a grain, most often corn, that with heat and pressure in a process known as extrusion is transformed into a variety of snackable shapes, from stars, to tubes, to the ever-popular curls (think Cheetos). The extruder settings can be adjusted to make the puffs crunchy for the adult palate or softer to be eaten safely by infants and young children. The most popular puffs are flavored with cheese, but there are many varieties, including those flavored (often minimally) with vegetables and fruits.

Because older children and adults love to snack on puffs and parents love them as infant finger food, global sales are expected to reach $31 billion by 2019. With that many puffs being extruded, you'd be correct if you guessed that there are a lot of puff manufacturers.

We spent days contacting puff manufacturers from coast to coast only to discover that their plants were all peanut-free, just as I had discovered with baby food manufacturers. Due to the high prevalence of food allergy, snack food manufacturers had segregated themselves more or less into two camps—those that make snacks with the Big Eight foods and those that would not allow most of the Big Eight foods on site. To be sure, there were some exceptions, such as cheese and wheat, but never peanut. Most manufacturers that make peanut snacks generally produce power bars and the like; many people with food allergies have to avoid many of these products. Puff manufacturers for the most part produce salty/crunchy snacks using fewer of the allergenic foods, so having additional food allergens on site would simply limit their market.

Producing our own peanut butter puff appeared to be another dead end. Scot knew a number of marketing people and lawyers who had some knowledge of food manufacture, so we turned to them for help. After a few brief conversations, we learned that we would need a business plan to have any hope of moving forward. Scot knows how to crunch numbers and I contributed my knowledge of some basic infant demographics and the pertinent medical information. With a business plan in hand, we engaged a law firm in Boston for further guidance. As luck would have it, our lawyer, Kurt, was a good friend of and counsel to a man named Rob, who had been a principal in a very successful snack food venture. He and his associates managed to create a new corn chip that became very popular. Anyone who could find success with yet another corn chip would certainly be able to help us create a great peanut food for infants.

It turns out that having a great new food idea might be a notion that perhaps too many people have and then set out to realize. While no one imagines they could practice medicine without going to medical school, we probably all know someone who has said something like, "Everyone loves my chocolate chip cookies, I think I should sell them." Kurt asked Rob to look at our business plan, but Rob knew all too well the barriers to starting any kind of food business. When he learned that a pediatrician and a business executive with a great idea but no food business experience had conceived this proposal, he knew everything he needed to know to decline the opportunity. We appealed to Kurt to persuade Rob to give us a shot. Rob relented; he would look at our plan, but only as a favor to Kurt.

Rob reviewed our plan and was blunt in his feedback:

Straight up[...]I have absolutely no interest in being involved in this concept beyond this email. I believe in being very truthful and direct and I mean no disrespect. I've taken three hours to write this for you to think about because Kurt is my friend. My apologies if it comes off negative[...]its meant to be honest[...]I'm sorry this is not a business or a business plan and it lacks depth and industry knowledge not to mention the business model has not been thought through in a thorough manner (you don't know what you don't know)[...]You have to re-educate an entire US society that children [infants] should eat peanut butter. Talk about a daunting task. *My overall recommendation: Don't waste your time, money, or family life, or career sacrifices on this endeavor.*

Scot and I found Rob's assessment harsh, unsympathetic, and completely without insight—how could he not see that this was in reality *a mission* articulated as a business plan? To be fair, it was also sobering and illuminating. A mission without the right map was not going to lead us to our goal.

We licked our wounds and resolved to redouble our efforts. If the barriers to manufacturing a new peanut food for infants were too great, perhaps we could instead find one. After all, in other countries infants ate peanut food; perhaps there was something better than Bamba out there already.

We found a number of peanut butter puffs from around the world, including several from Germany, Israel, and Bosnia. Unfortunately, none met our standards for nutrition and taste.

We considered the possibility that we would not find what we sought and it might be best to put our efforts into simply promoting Bamba. After all, the point was to promote the early introduction of peanut to infants along with a good way for infants to eat peanut food. Bamba was good—why let the perfect be the enemy of the good?

In July 2015, I stumbled upon a peanut butter puff I had somehow not previously found. Cheeky Monkey puffs were available in the U.S., but distribution was extremely limited and they had never caught on save for a tiny handful of fans. They were similar to Bamba in taste and appearance and also manufactured in Israel, but made of organic, non-GMO ingredients. They weren't perfect—they contained palm oil, had no whole grain, and would be better for infants if made with less salt—but they were a step in the right direction. Just days after discovering this product, I spoke with

Tzippi, an executive of the company, about promoting Cheeky Monkey in the U.S. as a great first peanut food for infants. She found fascinating the story about the prevalence of peanut allergy in the U.S., the study showing that peanut allergy could be prevented with early introduction, and the fact that the early introduction of peanut to infants in Israel had inspired the study. Practically on a whim, I was on a plane to Israel within a few days. With my office schedule completely booked, after an eleven-hour flight I had just two sweltering days to assess the potential of a possible collaboration. I engaged in long talks about puffs, peanuts, infants, and container ships with Tzippi and Yakov, a fruit and nut importer who had thoughts of investing in this project; saw the puffs in Israeli grocery stores; and ate a lot of falafel and hummus. We agreed that the possibilities were enticing and we would continue talking.

I came home aware of and intimidated by the enormous logistical and financial barriers to success in this venture. I had learned enough from my phone calls with local commercial kitchens and snack factories, my discussions with experts, my trip to Israel, and, yes, the dispiriting email from Rob, that this puzzle had a lot of pieces that I would have to fit together. But how could I fit together these puzzle pieces—finance, shipping, design, distribution, marketing, sales—when I barely recognized their shapes? And would the NIH and AAP, my fellow pediatric providers, and parents share my enthusiasm for early introduction?

CHAPTER V

The Guidelines for Introducing Peanut Food to Infants

"LEAP makes it clear that we can do something now to reverse the increasing prevalence of peanut allergy." (*NEJM* editorial 2/26/15, published concurrently with the LEAP study.)

"Look before you leap." (Samuel Butler)

"When it's time to leap ... leap, already." (Ron Sunog, MD)

THE GOAL OF LEAP WAS to answer the question "Does early introduction of peanut actually prevent peanut allergy?" The answer to the question would become useful only after the subsequent development of practical feeding guidelines pediatric providers could discuss with parents. With the LEAP conclusions published and the study results widely acknowledged as robust, no fewer than 10 authoritative medical organizations from the US, Canada, Europe, Australia, Israel, and Japan, comprised of leaders in pediatrics, allergy, immunology, and dermatology scrutinized the study. The reviewers from the AAP alone consisted of 11 primary contributors, five LEAP study contributors, and 28 secondary contributors, experts all.

Proceeding methodically, it wasn't until September 2015—seven full months after the study was published—that interim guidelines, "Consensus Communication on Early Peanut Introduction and the Prevention of Peanut Allergy in High-Risk Infants," were released by the American Academy of Pediatrics, with the promise of more extensive guidelines to follow within a year. These guidelines recommended that peanut be introduced to high-risk infants only, between four and six months of age, with the caveat that guidance by a physician might be beneficial.

Already convinced that Eat The Eight was the right approach, I was disappointed. Although I knew well the potential harm of overreach, I believed that beyond LEAP there was sufficient, if not conclusive, evidence to justify broader and more definitive recommendations. I would have to be patient and maintain optimism that the final guidelines would be more expansive.

Scot and I, our families vacationing together in Colorado when the interim guidelines were published, shared our disappointment. Scot remained steadfast in his conclusion that early introduction of peanut should be adopted for all infants, but grew concerned that this road would be far longer and bumpier then he had anticipated. Upon his return home later that month, he withdrew from Arachis to concentrate on his primary work and other ventures.

I called my friend Bob, a recently retired Healthcare CEO with endless enthusiasm and an indefatigable can-do attitude. Bob was interested in health, healthy eating, and finding a productive outlet for his energy. Also, he was a very new grandfather and the allergy prevention mission struck a chord. Bob was in.

By this time, I had entered into a partnership with Cheeky Monkey and, as luck would have it, just northwest of Boston a small, independent health food store with a long, hallowed history and devoted following, carried these puffs. Bob and I met there for a lunch of sprouty sandwiches and a planning session. The nuts and bolts of the planning were mundane and not worth recounting. Our conversation with the proprietor, Adam, on the other hand, was worth the price of lunch.

Adam said Cheeky Monkey was not enormously popular at his store, but there were a few customers who bought them on a regular basis. He allowed that he liked them quite a bit himself and even reported that one customer bought them as a snack for her dog because it was the dog's favorite organic treat. It turned out that Adam had a science background and I seized the opportunity to discuss infants and peanut allergy prevention with someone who understood nutritious food and science. Truth be told, by this time I was discussing this topic with anyone too polite to walk away. Scot had already christened me the peanut-for-infant evangelist and memorialized this by presenting me with a Superman T-shirt emblazoned with a large "E" in the center.

Adam listened studiously to my tale of infant feeding and food allergy, from the old advice, through a summary of the LEAP study and other evidence for early feeding of allergenic foods, to the denouement—promoting peanut butter puffs for infants. He agreed that the evidence was compelling and the mission to prevent peanut allergy laudable, but had concerns that his patrons might misinterpret the information. They might confuse the allergy prevention message with the idea that these puffs were to be used to treat peanut allergy, or feel somehow that his market was insensitive to children who had peanut allergy. Adam was sympathetic to the idea and the cause, but he envisioned irate customers complaining to the store manager. He offered moral support and allowed me to hand out my flyers, but he could not explicitly endorse my message.

In October 2015, I met Tzippi at Expo East, a natural foods exposition, in Baltimore. This event boasts almost 30,000 attendees, including sellers of natural foods from well-known brands and start-ups; buyers of these products, including stand-alone grocery stores and the largest chains in the country; and food distributors, advertisers, nutritionists, designers, investors, food bloggers, and media. Tzippi was there to provide samples to the buyers with the hope of finding new customers. I was happy to preach peanut allergy prevention and the nutritional virtues of peanut butter puffs.

Expo East did not lead to many orders, but had provided an opportunity to engage a broad cross section of people with different levels of knowledge about and perspectives on nutrition, food allergy, and appropriate infant feeding. It was now eight full months after the publication of LEAP and the extensive press coverage that "doctors had gotten it wrong and infants should have been eating peanut all along." Although encouraged by the interest in preventing peanut allergy with early introduction that was expressed by many I spoke with, nary a one could remember having previously heard this news. (I also heard the very occasional, unabashedly gleeful "I knew the doctors had it wrong!")

Over the next months, Bob and I did what little we could with the limited funds we had raised from our investors–the two of us. We contacted the handful of stores around the country that sold Cheeky Monkey and arranged in-store demos. But instead of food-sampling professionals, we hired nutritionists who understood and could teach shoppers about peanut allergy prevention and the early introduction of peanut food to infants. We supplied them with informational flyers that described the findings of LEAP and other studies, and also had catchy phrases like, "If you could give your infant a vaccine to prevent peanut allergy, you would. How about peanut butter puffs instead?"

At a dinner party in November I mentioned my peanut butter puff project to my friend Larry, a thoughtful psychiatrist with a very analytic mind and a fair amount of experience in the business world. To my surprise, he informed me that a decade earlier he had played a significant role in the success of a popular nutrition bar. He offered to provide guidance for my venture; I immediately created the position of company guru and appointed Larry to fill it.

The following month, we launched an effort to take what I had begun referring to as the "peanut allergy prevention project" directly to our most important audience--expectant parents and the parents of infants. We sent our puffs to Mom bloggers, engaged them to share our information with their readers, and sent cases of puffs to the lucky readers who won the bloggers' giveaway contests.

We also attended expos for expectant mothers and their partners in Boston, in December of 2015, and in Los Angeles, in March of 2016. Alongside the booths exhibiting strollers and high chairs with the latest fancy features, our offering was decidedly low-tech—a taste of peanut butter puffs along with literature about infant feeding. An impulsive taste of puffs before reading the ingredients was often followed by "That's funny tasting cheese," as the taste of peanut butter was wholly unexpected; ultimately, most liked the puffs. And although few could recite the entire list, most still believed that infants should avoid the Big Eight. Bob assisted me at these events. By March he was fully versed in the details of the discredited infant feeding guidelines, the sharp increase in the prevalence of food allergy, and the interim guidelines that were reason for hope. He was particularly enthusiastic in Los Angeles, as it was an excuse to visit family, especially his grandson, Jack. Jack was eight months old and Cheeky Monkey puffs were like catnip for him—he just couldn't get enough of them.

Meanwhile, additional evidence and opinion for early introduction of the Big Eight had continued to accumulate:

—At the American Academy of Allergy, Asthma, and Immunology Conference in Houston in February 2015, Dr. Gideon Lack recommended that infants not at high-risk, although not part of the LEAP study, be fed peanut products from four months of life.

—In November of 2015, the *Journal of the Canadian Medical Association* published a guideline for food introduction and allergy prevention in infants, stating "If a family asks how to prevent allergy in their children, our current advice is to introduce the allergenic foods at four to six months of age." This recommendation was based on a review of Canadian and American guidelines and more than 100 articles on allergy prevention with "the most robust level of evidence."

At the same time the LEAP study was underway, a group of researchers in London, including Dr. Lack of LEAP, were conducting the Enquiring About Tolerance (EAT) study. EAT investigated whether the early introduction of six allergenic foods (milk, peanut, sesame, fish, egg, wheat) to infants, while they continued breastfeeding, reduced the number who developed food allergies and other allergic diseases (such as eczema) by age three. In contrast to LEAP, EAT studied the early introduction of multiple allergenic foods rather than just peanut; infants were randomly chosen rather than limited to those at high-risk; and early introduction began as early as three months of age. While quite exceptional in its own right, the impact of this study was somewhat diminished by a lack of adherence to the feeding protocol by a significant number of infants. This produced results that after rigorous statistical analysis could provide only limited answers.

There was, in fact, a two-thirds reduction in overall food allergy among infants who consumed the recommended quantity of the allergenic foods, but because too few infants did so, this was not statistically significant. The reduction in food allergy was greatest for peanut and egg. It was also found that there was more protection associated with consuming larger amounts of the foods for a longer duration.

Why some families did not adhere to the feeding regimen was uncertain, but it was suggested that additional support to parents for early introduction might have been helpful.

Food Standards Agency, an independent government department of the UK dedicated to food safety and public health, concluded that The EAT Study found that early introduction of the allergenic foods into the infant diet might be effective in food allergy prevention and that this approach was safe.

In May of 2016, results of the Canadian Healthy Infant Longitudinal Study (CHILD) *unequivocally supported the Eat The Eight concept.* That study found that the early introduction of solid foods and an increased diversity of allergenic foods reduced the risk of sensitization to food. The authors concluded that this reaffirmed *"the paradigm shift from delayed food introduction and food avoidance to earlier introduction of diverse foods for allergy prevention"* (italics mine). Maxwell Tran, the lead investigator at McMaster University in Hamilton, Ontario, Canada stated, "The clinical implications of our findings are that early introduction of allergenic foods (egg, cow's milk products, and peanut) before age one should be encouraged and is better than food avoidance for reducing the risk of food sensitization [...]"

That same month, the Australasian Society of Clinical Immunology and Allergy published new comprehensive infant feeding and allergy prevention guidelines based on current published evidence and the consensus of participants in an Infant Feeding Summit hosted by the Centre for Food and Allergy Research in May 2016. A key recommendation of the report was, *"All infants should be given allergenic solid foods including peanut butter, cooked egg, dairy and wheat products in the first year of life. This includes infants at high risk of allergy"* (italics mine).

While immersed in promoting the early introduction of peanut, I remained convinced of the importance of early introduction of the Big Eight and had never stopped contemplating ways to promote this. My experiences at the food and Mom's expos and discussions with the various marketing people I had encountered over the previous months had helped me understand in a profound way that we live in an Instagram world. A message to parents would have to be short and sweet—catchy, easy to digest in just a few seconds, and memorable. Inspired by the phrase "Back To Sleep," I coined "Eat The Eight." I then hired a talented local designer to translate my vision into an image, which resulted in the birth of my "eight-fant."

From that time on, when talking about peanut allergy prevention I made sure to present the broader message to Eat The Eight. Our small team persevered through the summer and into fall, handing out puffs and literature at various events. But by the time the last leaves of red and gold had fallen off the trees, Larry was advising me to throw in the towel. He remained supportive of the mission, but ever the faithful advisor he had analyzed the viability of the venture through clear eyes, not filtered through the prism of optimism I peered through. He had concluded that without a lot of cash, which it was clear we could not raise, we could neither succeed with Cheeky Monkey nor get meaningful attention for Eat The Eight.

Late December of 2016, I closed the Cheeky Monkey Corporation. My Eat The Eight discussions would be limited to counseling parents at office visits. It was still unknown when the NIH would publish the definitive new guidelines for infant feeding or what they would be.

In January of 2017, just days after filing papers to officially close Cheeky Monkey, Inc., the NIH released the Addendum Guidelines (so called because they were intended as an addendum to the NIH infant feeding guidelines published in 2010) for the introduction of peanut to infants:

—Children with severe eczema, egg allergy, or both: Strongly consider evaluation with peanut-specific IgE and/or skin prick test and, if necessary, an oral food challenge. Based on test results, introduce peanut-containing foods at four to six months of age.

—Children with mild to moderate eczema: Introduce peanut containing foods at around six months of age.

—Children with no eczema or any food allergy: Introduce peanut containing foods at an appropriate age and in accordance with family preferences and cultural practices.

After a wait of nearly two full years for the final guidelines, I was again disappointed. I had expected recommendations that would more enthusiastically urge parents to feed peanut to all infants early and often. And despite the mounting evidence from other studies that could well support a campaign for early introduction of all the allergenic foods, there was not even a rumor that such guidelines were under consideration.

The Addendum Guidelines were disappointing, but ironically, I felt more strongly that it was not yet time to quit Eat The Eight. Based on what then transpired, I would suggest the fates agreed.

In January 2017, Larry discovered Puffworks, a new company that manufactured peanut butter puffs in Portland, Oregon. Although with the demise of Cheeky Monkey he had retired from this

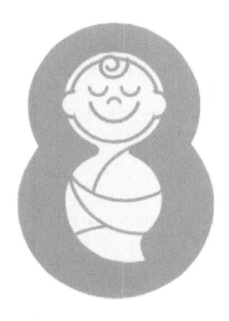

EIGHTFANT

endeavor, his curiosity got the better of him and he called the founder. Rich, a quirky, rough-around-the-edges guy who had experienced some business setbacks but had a no-quit attitude, had discovered Bamba while working in Israel for a few years. Upon his return to Portland, he decided that the U.S. needed better-for-you peanut butter puffs that were made right here at home—and he was going to make them. He had run into the same barriers to manufacture that I had, so he arranged to have unflavored puffs manufactured to his specifications and shipped to him. He then completed their transformation into peanut butter puffs in his basement, which he had converted into a small food manufacturing facility. (Why hadn't I thought of that?) Having reached the limits of his manufacturing capacity, he had been talking with Greg, a talented CEO with food industry experience, about working together to get to the next level—wider distribution of the best puff they could make.

Larry put me in touch with Rich and Greg. Already committed to the concept of a very nutritious snack food, they were immediately intrigued by the idea of adding peanut allergy prevention to the company mission; I was welcomed on board as Medical Advisor. I also sacrificed my midlife-crisis sports car fund to invest in the company.

As we turned our attention to the details of making the best peanut butter puff specifically formulated for infants, we discussed puff texture, the amount of peanut protein, and the feasibility of making the product organic and using whole grain corn. I learned that the logistics of creating this kind of product are not simple, from sourcing organic ingredients, to controlling costs in order to keep the product affordable, to getting the extruder settings right for whole grain. (Most extruded puffs—including all other peanut butter puffs—are made of refined grain. Getting this part of the operation right required consultation with the high mavens of extrusion technology.)

Along with getting the formula for Puffworks baby right, it was clear to the team that it made sense to transition the entire line of Puffworks puffs to organic, non-GMO, and mostly whole-grain. With the help of Guru Hari's research and development, Jack's design work, and Holly's marketing, Puffworks recently completed production of our first batch of these nutritious snacks.

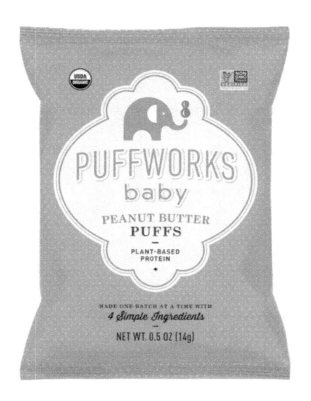

PUFFWORKS baby

CHAPTER VI

Going Beyond the Guidelines

Cost-benefit analysis: "[...] a systematic approach to estimate the strengths and weaknesses of alternatives[...]a systematic process for calculating and comparing benefits and costs of a decision [...]" (Wikipedia)

Pascal's Wager: "Even under the assumption that God's existence is unlikely, the potential benefits of believing are so vast as to make betting on theism rational."

(Pascal's Wager, the Internet Encyclopedia of Philosophy)

THE LEAP STUDY WAS PUBLISHED in February of 2015, after which panels of experts deliberated for almost two years before publishing the Addendum Guidelines. In October 2017, fully 10 months after the Addendum Guidelines were established, only 11% of pediatricians had integrated them into practice. Perhaps this should be unsurprising, as studies have shown that physicians are not immune to the inclination to cling to obsolete information. A study in 2017 demonstrated that pediatricians continued to use established treatments even after they had been discredited by new research. Dr. Aaron Carroll, Professor of Pediatrics at Indiana University School of Medicine, attributes this to the difficulty they have "unlearning things."

If medical providers failed to adopt the Guidelines, there would be little influence on parents and little change in how infants are fed. Broader guidelines might inspire more robust action, but the evidence from LEAP was limited to peanuts and high-risk infants, and history had shown that making unsupported recommendations could be costly.

Despite this, it is my contention that the Addendum Guidelines are too conservative and restrained and that careful weighing of all considerations would endorse early introduction of all Big Eight foods to all infants. And it appears that a number of leading experts wholeheartedly agree:

—"My clinical approach has long favored early peanut introduction [...] *For low-risk infants, I encourage home-based introduction of peanut (not as whole nuts)"* (italics mine). Dr. George Du Toit, lead LEAP investigator, *NEJM* online forum, 2/25/15.

—"[...] studies have very consistently shown that early introduction is the way to go[...]now we say, 'Give foods early.'" Dr. Jonathon Spergel, Chief of the Allergy Section at Children's Hospital of Philadelphia, "Delay Food Introduction to Prevent Food Allergy? It Doesn't Work," *Medscape Editorial*, 5/2015.

—"Early introduction in this group [low-risk], *though not emphasized in the guidelines, should contribute to lower overall rate of peanut allergy*" (italics mine). Dr. James R. Baker, Jr., FARE CEO, Food Allergy Research and Education, Webinar, 1/2017.

—"Infants without eczema or any other food allergy aren't likely to develop an allergy to peanuts. *To be on the safe side, it's still a good idea for them to start eating peanuts from an early age*" (italics mine). Dr. Francis Collins, Director of the NIH, "Peanut Allergy: Early Exposure is Key to Prevention," NIH Director's Blog, 1/10/2017.

—"*Have infants eat allergenic foods early and have them eat these foods often*" (italics mine). Dr. David M. Fleischer, an author of the Addendum Guidelines, "Guidelines for Life After LEAP," *Contemporary Pediatrics*, 4/3/2017.

All of these recommendations—from experts that include the Chief of Pediatric Allergy at one of the nation's leading children's hospitals; the CEO of a prominent allergy education and research institution; a LEAP study lead investigator; a Director of the National Institute of

Health; and an allergist who contributed his expertise to promulgating the Guidelines—go beyond the Addendum Guidelines. Are they reckless or is there more to the equation than just the concrete evidence from the LEAP study?

Evidence Based Medicine can tell us how good a study was, how strong and reliable the evidence is. The Addendum Guidelines generally reflect adherence to EBM standards. Making a decision about the best course of action when starting infants on solid foods, on the other hand, is not so simple and we must take context into account. The context missing from the Addendum Guidelines is the cost benefit analysis. And, similar to Pascal's wager, it can be shown that the potential benefits of early introduction are so vast and the cost so low, it's the correct approach, even if, much like the existence of God, it hasn't been proven beyond any doubt. (This is not to be interpreted as advocating for or against the existence of God, as this is far beyond the scope of *Eat The Eight* and far outside my field of expertise.)

Researchers have analyzed EBM in order to determine how best to use it in medical decision making. One evaluation concluded that evidence-based recommendations *are more useful when taking into account the benefits and harms* of health interventions and that science and evidence need to be tempered by clinical acumen. Another suggested that there are actually *two different kinds of EBM*: one, which the authors called epistemological EBM, focuses solely on the strength of knowledge derived from clinical trials; the other, which they referred to as practical EBM, describes the best way to practice medicine. The expert recommendations I quoted

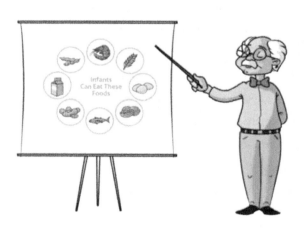

EXPERT ADVICE

are the inevitable result of the official guidelines tempered by clinical acumen, which might also be described as deriving practical **EBM** from epistemological **EBM**. I would suggest this application of clinical acumen to the findings of the LEAP study, in order to find the best way to practice medicine, is an example of what we mean when we use the term "the art of medicine."

The Safety of Early Introduction

At a recent visit in my office, I discussed starting solid foods with Jennifer, four-month-old Ali's Mom. Ali was her first and she had not previously thought much about how to go about this, but she did remember having read and heard a few things about infant feeding. Although uncertain about infant feeding guidelines, she was pretty sure that the idea of feeding her infant peanut food, eggs, and fish made her uncomfortable. Jennifer suggested it might be difficult for her to make the active decision to incorporate these foods into Ali's diet, so she would "decide to not decide" and simply avoid these foods. Of course, "not deciding" is tantamount to deciding against early introduction, and decisions have consequences.

A parent has only two choices: either introduce the Big Eight early or delay introduction. Although the LEAP study looked only at high-risk infants and peanut, this decision must still be made for all infants and all of the Big Eight. Despite the lack of incontrovertible proof that early introduction of the Big Eight prevents food allergy:

—We know that the practice of delaying these foods coincided with a sharp increase in the prevalence of food allergy in children.

—We know that there is no harm from early introduction.

—We know that in Israel the practice of early introduction of peanut is directly related to a lower prevalence of peanut allergy than in countries that practiced delayed introduction. (There are also other countries in Africa and Asia that practice early introduction and also have a lower prevalence of peanut allergy.)

—And we have the LEAP study results, which showed that early introduction of peanut is clearly beneficial for high-risk infants.

We can therefore safely conclude that for all infants, not only does delayed introduction not decrease the risk of developing food allergy, but early introduction is at the very least no worse and *is likely better* in this regard.

Ali's mother was receptive to this explanation and upon reconsideration concluded that it made sense for Ali to Eat the Eight.

But is the fact that early introduction is *likely* better with regard to developing food allergy reason enough to recommend it? Are there other risks or costs to consider? And is the potential benefit sufficient to outweigh the risks and costs?

Potential for Effect on Infant Nutrition

Over my years in practice, I have seen the number of mothers devoted to breastfeeding increase. Ali's mother wondered if trying to introduce peanut food and the Big Eight might somehow interfere with breastfeeding. Fortunately, LEAP researchers anticipated possible concern about potential adverse effects of early introduction on infant nutrition. They evaluated the diet and growth of the infants in the LEAP study and found that there had been no effect on the duration of breastfeeding and no negative impact on growth or nutrition.

The EAT study also investigated this concern and similarly concluded that the early introduction of allergenic foods (not just peanut) did not affect breastfeeding.

These findings were of no little importance because some breastfeeding advocates, including the World Health Organization (WHO), stringently support breastfeeding exclusively until the age of six months based on the concern that starting solids early might hasten weaning, thereby depriving the infant of the full advantages of breastfeeding. The Australian Breastfeeding Association has pointed out that when introducing solids, nutritional issues, risk of illness, risk of adverse effect on breastfeeding, and developmental readiness needs to be considered in addition to concerns about developing food allergy. They note also that despite some studies suggesting that earlier is better (for allergy prevention), there is no strong evidence that early introduction at four months is superior to early introduction at six months.

Another study suggested that a compromise to recommend solid food introduction at around six months but not before four months, as recommended in the recently published Australasian guidelines, could satisfy both allergy prevention and breastfeeding concerns.

On balance, the studies have been reassuring that early introduction of allergenic foods can be achieved without adverse effect on infant nutrition. Ali could Eat The Eight and there would be no effect on her breastfeeding.

Relation of Age of Child to Severity of Allergic Reaction

Leanne, a nurse in my office, brought her daughter, Franny, to see me and when we discussed the early introduction of the Big Eight she well understood that an allergic reaction could occur at any age. Still, she wondered, "What if Franny had a reaction and it were worse for her at six months than it might be if she were to have the same reaction at 15 months or three years of age?" As a nurse in my office, she's had the experience of ushering a child having an allergic reaction to food into a room to be quickly evaluated; the image of something similar happening to Franny made her quite anxious.

As I described in Chapter II, allergic reactions to food are variable and range from mild rash to anaphylaxis and even death. Even if early introduction results in fewer children who develop food allergy, some number of infants will have an allergic reaction.

What if Leanne's concern is valid and reactions to food are more severe for infants than for older children?

Although anaphylaxis can occur at any age and information about anaphylaxis in infants is mixed, studies generally conclude that it is less common in infancy than in later childhood. A study from 2001 showed that of 32 fatal cases that had been reported to a national registry, none were younger than two years of age. A review of emergency room cases from 2011 found that 29% who developed anaphylaxis were age two years or younger, but did not specify how many of these children were under one year of age. A review of a pediatric allergy database published in 2013 found that infant anaphylaxis accounted for about 22% of cases, while another review from Europe in 2016 found that fewer than 1% with anaphylaxis were less than one year of age. Clearly, the precise rate of anaphylaxis in infants is difficult to ascertain, but appears to be significantly lower than the rate in older children.

One way to put this into perspective is to realize that *new foods are introduced to infants and children all the time, there is always some risk of a reaction, yet no screening tests for allergy are contemplated, much less actually done, before feeding an infant a new food.* One study even questioned the utility of screening high-risk infants prior to the introduction of peanut (which the interim guidelines recommend ought to be considered, but not required, for high-risk infants) by pointing out this very fact. Another study done in 2017 to evaluate how early introduction of peanut might effect a large population (rather than an individual infant) noted that a first exposure to foods within the first 12 months of life is rarely fatal and that there have actually been no deaths reported related to peanut exposure within the first year of life. Another study from 2016 looked at the possible implications of early peanut exposure and noted that among both low- and high-risk infants whose parents chose to introduce peanut at home in the first year of life and also in 150 peanut-allergic infants undergoing hospital based peanut challenge, there had been no life threatening reactions.

Leanne's concern is valid and the thought of one's infant having an anaphylactic reaction is distressing. Yet despite there being no doubt that some infants will experience allergic reactions to food and some of these reactions will be severe, *infants are less likely than older children to have the most severe or life-threatening reactions.*

It has been suggested that an additional benefit of early introduction might be a lower risk of missing an allergic reaction. Amal Assa'ad, MD, Associate Director, Division of Allergy and Immunology of the Cincinnati Children's Hospital Medical Center and an author of the Addendum Guidelines stated, "Food allergy reactions are immediate, so if a mother is in her own home, and she gives her baby that first bit of peanut butter and they react, she is going to know, and she is going to take that child to the doctor. If we leave children to their own devices, and someone in daycare gives them a peanut butter sandwich, they may have a reaction, and no one will notice." The higher likelihood of a mild reaction being observed would result in a lower risk of eating that food again, thereby reducing the risk of a more significant reaction in the future.

Although a reaction during infancy is a risk of early introduction, *it is almost certainly less of a risk* than later introduction of the food.

Early introduction of the Big Eight poses *no cost in terms of additional health risk.* This provides solid support for the claim by David Fleischer, MD, Associate Professor of Pediatrics and Associate Medical Director of the Children's Hospital Colorado Research Institute, that "data at this time demonstrate *there is no reason to delay the introduction of any food, including all highly allergenic foods, into an infant's diet beyond 4 to 6 months of age.*" (italics mine)

Potential For Benefit

The goal of early introduction of the Big Eight to infants is to decrease the number of children who develop food allergy, which would result in benefits to the child, their family, and society. The burdens of food allergy were described in Chapter II; just how much could they be mitigated?

We know that high-risk infants who eat peanut stand to benefit enormously, as LEAP showed that with early introduction to these infants, peanut allergy would be prevented in over 80%. How much additional benefit might there be, however, if early introduction guidelines for peanut were expanded to all infants?

To begin with, it is a safe assumption that some infants who are in fact high-risk are simply not recognized as such by their parents and would, therefore, potentially miss the benefits of early introduction. Emphasizing the recommendation for all infants would decrease the possibility that these infants would miss early introduction inadvertently. So, we could expect a reduction of over 80% in the development of peanut allergy in infants who are high-risk, but have been erroneously identified as not high-risk.

It is also known that some infants who don't fit LEAP high-risk criteria for peanut allergy—specifically, having egg allergy and/or severe eczema—are at increased risk due to other factors. For example, an infant with a sibling who has peanut allergy has a 7% risk of developing peanut allergy compared to the overall 2.5% rate of peanut allergy in children. Again, these infants might benefit from early introduction, but their parents might intentionally keep peanut from them and possibly miss an opportunity to decrease their risk of developing peanut allergy.

Further, the Canadian Pediatric Society has noted that the definition of high risk is blurred by a lack of international consensus. The traditional definition of high risk for developing food allergy in general (including, but not limited to, peanut allergy) is a positive family history of eczema, food allergy, allergic rhinitis, and/or asthma, and numerous other factors are currently under investigation. It also stands to reason that individual risk lies on a continuum for all of these factors and does not fit neatly into high, medium, and low categories. If an infant has risk factors, it would seem prudent to pursue any available intervention that *might* reduce risk, *when there is no cost to the intervention.* One can only speculate as to the number of cases of food allergy that could be prevented.

To be clear, it has not been proven that early introduction would benefit those with risk factors for food allergy other than those identified in the LEAP study (egg allergy and/or severe eczema). But, for example, a similar strategy can be seen in recommendations for reducing the risk of cardiovascular disease. My father-in-law's cardiologist has long recommended that he exercise to reduce his risk for cardiovascular disease, despite the fact that both his parents had cardiovascular disease and little was known about the efficacy of this recommendation in this setting. It wasn't until April 2018 that Stanford researchers published an observational study of almost a half-million people, which showed an association between high fitness levels and low heart disease, even among those at genetic risk. The senior author of the study pointed out that both those with low and high genetic risk should exercise because health is influenced by a mix of genes and the environment. The same is almost certainly true regarding the development of food allergy.

It is also quite certain that limiting a strong early introduction recommendation of peanut to only infants defined as high-risk by LEAP misses many infants who ultimately develop peanut allergy, because a simple analysis shows that *many children who develop peanut allergy must come from the moderate- and low-risk groups.*

With 2.5% of children now peanut allergic, we can estimate that of the 4,000,000 infants born annually, 100,000 will develop peanut allergy in the absence of early introduction. (Given the trend, the actual number could be higher.) Determining exactly how many infants are high-, medium-, and low-risk is difficult and uncertain, but using available data, I have calculated that only 120,000 of the

4,000,000 infants meet high-risk criteria. (For those with an interest in the wonkish math, my complete calculations are in the next chapter.) Absent early introduction of peanut, these 120,000 infants would yield 29,000 cases of peanut allergy. That leaves 3,880,000 infants who are medium- and low-risk, from which the remaining 71,000 new cases of peanut allergy annually—61,000 from the medium-risk group and 10,000 from the low-risk—must come. One report, using data from the HealthNuts study (a comprehensive food allergy study performed by the Murdoch Children's Research Institute), puts the annual number of peanut allergy cases from the low-risk group even higher, at 23% of all cases. *In other words, around 71% of infants who develop peanut allergy would not be identified as high-risk by LEAP study criteria.* Further, if early introduction benefits only high-risk infants, so few infants would avoid peanut allergy that we would still have a rather sizable peanut allergy problem. The extremely low rate of peanut allergy in Israel, where early introduction is practiced, would seem to indicate that early introduction almost certainly benefits medium- and low-risk infants.

Early introduction to high-risk infants, by preventing 80% (low estimate based on LEAP) of peanut allergy cases, would prevent 23,200 cases of peanut allergy. How effective early introduction would be for the infants not at high-risk is unknown; however, the potential benefit is great as this group accounts for about 2.5 times as many cases of peanut allergy as the high-risk group. If early introduction were only half as effective in this group, about 28,000 cases of peanut allergy would be prevented—over 20% *more* cases than would be prevented by early introduction in the high-risk group.

This has to be considered in the context that there is no risk to early introduction.

How much additional benefit might there be by expanding early introduction recommendations from just peanut to the Big Eight? The burden of food allergy is well known, but as we see, exactly how much this could be reduced by early introduction is unknowable. At the same time, with no cost to the early introduction of the Big Eight, *any* benefit would be valuable and meaningful.

From a financial perspective, if early introduction were applied only to peanut and high-risk infants, at approximately 23,000 cases of peanut allergy prevented and a savings of approximately $4,000 per case (the average additional annual medical expense borne by the family of a child with food allergy), there would be an annual savings of $92,000,000 nationally. Even at a cost of several hundred dollars per case for a visit to the allergist and allergy testing prior to feeding peanut (the Addendum Guidelines recommend that this should be considered), we can estimate a total annual savings of about $80,000,000.

With 4,000,000 infants born annually and a current prevalence of food allergy of about 8% of children, we can predict that about 320,000 will develop food allergy. Even if early introduction is effective in preventing only 10% of them from developing food allergy—far lower than the greater than 80% reduction experienced by high-risk infants in the LEAP study—the savings would be an additional $128,000,000. As all of these children can be fed the Big

Eight without prior evaluation—no medical costs—$128,000,000 represents net savings.

Of note, if food allergy prevention could be successfully implemented in low-income families, the savings would be even greater. Food allergy prevalence is greater among the poor and they incur 2.5 times the hospitalization costs of higher-income children (thought to be the result of less access to specialists, medications, and allergen-free foods).

The number of lives saved by early introduction of the Big Eight is more difficult to calculate, as estimates of deaths due to anaphylaxis from food range from about 10 to 200 annually. A reduction in food allergy prevalence of 10% would presumably lead to an equivalent reduction in deaths, approximately 1-20 lives saved annually.

The precise number of children who would benefit from early introduction of the Big Eight is unknown. On the other hand, it is quite likely that some (in addition to those at high-risk for peanut allergy to whom peanut is introduced early) would benefit and this would result in a significant return on investment, no matter how little the return, as there is no cost.

In addition to the zero cost and the vast potential benefits I already noted, there would be ancillary nutritional benefits.

I am very familiar with the typical infant diet and know well that it can be improved. The Big Eight foods as a whole are very nutritious. Well-known pediatrician, author, and spokesperson for the AAP, Dr. Tanya Altmann recommends eggs, fish, dairy, and nuts (not as whole nuts) as four of the 'Eleven Essential Foods' to feed infants in her book, *What to Feed Your Baby.*

A nutritious diet is defined both by the foods that are eaten and the foods that are avoided. Adding new nutritious foods to infants' diets would make it easier to eliminate less nutritious foods, perhaps beginning with white rice. In 2011 Dr. Alan Greene started the WhiteOut movement to promote a better diet for infants. As Dr. Greene put it, "It's no wonder that America's kids are hooked on junk food. For the past 50 years the majority of babies in the United States have been given white rice cereal for their very first bite of solid food. Metabolically, it's similar to eating sugar. White rice cereal is the number one source of food calories for most babies until about 11 months old." His goal was to end the tradition of white rice cereal as baby's first food—a 50-year-old tradition at the time WhiteOut was started in 2010—in one year. There has been some improvement, but that goal remains elusive even now, eight years later. Expanding infants' menu with the Big Eight foods might very well help.

It has also been reported that junk food habits often start by nine months of age; by one year of age, diets often contain excessive amounts of sugar and salt. In June 2018, a paper presented at a meeting of the American Society for Nutrition supported this, noting that infants and toddlers aged 6-23 months consumed an average of 4.2 teaspoons of sugar daily. To put this in perspective, the American Heart Association recommends that adult women consume no more than six teaspoons of added sugar daily. Infants and young children are more likely to accept a greater variety of foods and flavors with repeated exposure and eating the Eight early and often would result in a more varied and nutritious diet from the time an infant starts solids. Studies show that early consumption of nutritious foods leads to a greater likelihood that children will prefer these foods and also that healthier eating patterns will persist in later childhood.

The cost benefit analysis of a universal recommendation to Eat The Eight falls overwhelmingly on the side of recommendation. Further evidence would help replace speculation with facts and there are some additional studies being done, but the economics of research means that we should expect additional research in this area to be limited, because it has very little commercial value and is often dependent on increasingly scarce government funding. We must, therefore, make our best decision using the information at hand. (As you will see in Chapter VIII, despite the reality that the findings of the LEAP study do not lend themselves easily to medicalization and monetization, that does not mean there aren't those who will try—peanut pills anyone?)

Again, many experts have come to this very same conclusion. At the American College of Asthma, Allergy, and Immunology meeting in San Francisco in November 2016, Dr. Katie Allen, pediatric gastroenterologist and allergist and Theme Director of Population Health and Group Leader of Gastro and Food Allergy at Murdoch Children's Research Institute, gave a presentation titled "Results From the LEAP Study Should Be Applied to Food Other Than [Just] Peanut." The first slide from her presentation provides an apt summary:

—LEAP provides the first RCT [randomized control trial] evidence that delaying the introduction of peanut increases peanut allergy

—There is a growing body of observational and trial data for other foods (including egg) that delaying the introduction of allergenic solids increases the risk of food allergy

—Recent systematic review now available synthesizing these findings

—The timing of changes to infant feeding guidelines mirrors the rise in incidence of food allergy

—Even if these findings are due to reverse causation—*i.e. those at highest risk of food allergy are the ones most likely to avoid allergenic foods such as peanut, egg and cow's milk*—timely introduction won't be harmful

—Babies don't read guidelines—they eat when they are ready

—*Conclusion: We should uniformly recommend that allergenic solids should not be delayed and should be introduced in the first year of life* (italics mine)

CHAPTER VII

Peanut Allergy Risk Calculation

THERE ARE 4,000,000 INFANTS BORN in the US annually.

The most recent research shows that ~2.5% of children have peanut allergy.

We can expect 100,000 (2.5% of 4,000,000) of these infants to develop peanut allergy (in the absence of early introduction of peanut).

(2.5% is the current prevalence, but with the prevalence known to have been growing for years the number of new cases annually would be higher than 2.5%. Conversely, some experts suggest that parents over-report peanut allergy. Given this, it seems that 2.5% is a reasonable working estimate.)

Prevalence of Eczema and Egg Allergy

12.97% of children have eczema, 7% of these children with eczema have severe eczema. Therefore, 0.9% of children have severe eczema (7% of the 12.97%) and ˜12% have mild to moderate eczema (93% of the 12.97%).

2% (at most) of children have egg allergy.

High-Risk

Assuming approximately the same eczema and egg allergy prevalence for infants as for children, ˜3% of infants are high-risk = **120,000 infants annually** (3% of 4,000,000). (This number is likely somewhat lower as the two groups—infants with eczema and infants with egg allergy—overlap, which would result in less than 3% in total.)

Moderate-Risk

12% of children have mild or moderate eczema = **480,000 infants annually** (12% of 4,000,000).

Low-Risk

All the rest = **3,400,000 infants annually**

The **LEAP** study found that of the initial cohort of high-risk infants (716), 10.6% (76) were determined to be already peanut allergic based on the skin prick test. 13.7% (44) in the peanut avoidance group (321) developed peanut allergy.

Taken together, 24.3% of high-risk infants will develop peanut allergy.

If **24.3% of high-risk infants** develop peanut allergy, **high-risk infants** account for ˜29,000 of the total of 100,000 who will develop peanut allergy annually.

The remaining 71,000 cases of peanut allergy come from the moderate- and low-risk groups. Moderate-risk infants have six times the risk of low-risk infants.

Moderate-risk infants then account for 6/7 of 71,000 = ˜61,000 annually.

Low-risk infants then account for 1/7 of 71,000 = ˜10,000 annually.

CHAPTER VIII

Do Good or Do No Harm

"The physician must [...] have two special objects in view with regard to disease, namely, to do good or to do no harm."

(Hippocrates, Father of Medicine)

MY ANALYSIS HAS SHOWN THAT with allergy prevention benefits (some certain, some potential), additional health benefits, and no cost, the value of early introduction of the Big Eight is significant. Yet there are no official guidelines from the NIH or AAP that make this recommendation and physicians have been slow to adopt the limited guidelines that prevail. Is it possible that despite the very strong evidence of LEAP, the suggestive evidence of other studies, and the extremely favorable cost-benefit equation, the standard for making an Eat The Eight recommendation has not been met? To provide perspective and help answer this question we can look at a broad variety of other medical conditions, the accepted and standard treatments for these conditions, and the level of support provided by evidence and cost-benefit analysis for these treatments.

Comparison to a Vaccine

Meningitis is an infection of the brain and spinal cord membranes that can be caused by a number of different germs. Meningococcal meningitis is a rare but potentially very devastating form of this disease for which a vaccine was approved in 2004. About 80% of teenagers have had their first dose of the two dose series. (I refer here to a vaccine that protects against four of the five most invasive serogroups of meningococcus. A second vaccine, covering only the fifth serogroup was approved in 2014 and is now also recommended and routinely administered starting at age 16, but for simplicity's sake I have not included in this comparison information about the second vaccine.) The overall incidence of infection is fewer than two per million; the incidence for the 16-23 year old age group is about three per million. Although rare, even if diagnosis is timely and treatment is appropriate, 10-15% of those infected will die and 10-20% will suffer extremely serious complications that can include brain damage, kidney damage, deafness, and loss of a limb.

A study published in 2005 evaluated how many lives would be saved by the vaccine and at what cost. It revealed that vaccination of all 11-year-olds (the first shot of a two shot series is routinely given at age 11) would prevent 270 cases of meningococcal disease and 36 deaths over a 22-year period, which would be a 46% decrease in the expected burden of disease. Given the cost of paying for and administering the vaccine and taking into account both the savings realized from medical costs these protected children would not incur and the additional productivity to society their good health would allow, the net cost to society for adolescents would be

$633,000 per meningococcal case prevented and $121,000 per life-year (a single year of good health) saved.

This example indicates that when a treatment can prevent significant morbidity and mortality, it is generally recommended by experts and providers and welcomed by parents, even when the total number who will benefit is small (in this case because the disease is rare) and the cost is high. Whether the benefits are worth the cost in a world of resources that are not infinite is a debate worthy of philosophers, politicians, and public health policy makers. In practice, it is the Advisory Committee on Immunization Practices (ACIP) that makes this evaluation and advises the Center for Disease Control and Prevention (CDC). As it stands, the CDC recommends the vaccine (it is not required) for all 11-year-olds and pediatricians in general follow this. (Debate of value aside, I have diagnosed and treated meningococcal meningitis and am grateful for the availability of a vaccine that I routinely recommend and administer to my patients.)

Even if limited to exactly the narrow population of high-risk infants as studied in LEAP, early introduction of peanut would prevent around 23,200 cases of peanut allergy annually—*at a net annual savings of around $80,000,000, rather than any cost at all.* This would pay for a meningitis vaccine series for about 320,000 11-year-olds. There can be little doubt that a recommendation that all infants Eat The Eight would result in even more net benefit. *If early introduction of the allergenic foods prevented only two deaths annually, it would compare favorably with the meningococcal vaccine.*

Comparison to a Surgical Procedure

Having to decide what to recommend using only information that is not definitive is hardly unique to determining infant feeding guidelines. Expanding the recommendation of the LEAP study to Eat The Eight for all infants generates no cost. What cost do we accept for a surgical procedure with questionable efficacy?

Consider arthroscopic partial menisectomy (APM), a common knee surgery for age-related degenerative knee problems, which accounted for two-thirds of all arthroscopic knee procedures on elderly patients in 2016. A tear of the cartilage of the knee (the meniscus), due to degeneration with age, is present in 67% of people over 65 years old who have no symptoms of knee pain and in 91% of those who do have symptoms. Surgical procedures to treat this condition have been performed for more than 100 years. Initially, this consisted of removal of the cartilage in its entirety based on the belief, without evidence, that once removed, the cartilage could no longer cause symptoms. It turned out that with time most of these post-surgical knees (now absent cartilage) got worse, developing significant arthritis (inflammation of the joint). (Does this story have familiar echoes?) With time, surgeons began to remove just the damaged cartilage, rather than all of it. There continued to be limited evidence that the more limited procedure was beneficial, yet with the advent of arthroscopy—a less invasive procedure making the surgery less risky and recovery easier—the number of these procedures performed grew, so that today the most common orthopedic procedure in the US is arthroscopy to remove damaged cartilage in the knee joint. *700,000 such procedures are performed annually at a cost of four billion dollars.* In other words, as the intervention became easier to implement (less invasive surgery), the number of procedures performed grew, at enormous cost, despite a lack of good evidence of benefit. In fact, the most recent studies suggest that this procedure is greatly overused and in many cases no better than sham surgery or physical therapy.

This is not to say that menisectomy is never of benefit, only that we are unable at this time to determine with certainty who would benefit and who would not. (Some experts suggest that the surgery is of benefit to repair cartilage damaged by injury—the minority of cases—rather than age-related wear and tear and they recommend the procedure be limited to these cases, but that is not the standard currently adhered to by many orthopedic surgeons.) In contrast to this, if Eat The Eight were universally recommended, to both those who would benefit and those who only might benefit, at best far fewer children would develop food allergy. At worst, infants' diets would be improved *at no cost*—a bargain, to say the least.

Comparison to Antibiotic Treatment of an Infection

When attempting to calculate the potential benefit of recommending that all infants Eat The Eight, it is known that not all infants will benefit. After all, early introduction of peanut resulted in benefit for 'only' about 80% of high-risk infants in LEAP. Is there a minimum threshold for how many are expected to benefit in order to recommend an intervention?

Last winter, I sent three-year-old Ethan to the hospital to be admitted for pneumonia. As per standard protocol, antibiotics were started as soon as possible upon his arrival. This despite the likelihood that his infection, like that of most children hospitalized with pneumonia, was caused by a virus, a germ that doesn't respond to antibiotics. Antibiotics have a financial cost and the risk of side effects. Further, it is well known that the overuse of antibiotics is at a crisis level, having led to an increase in the presence of bacteria that are resistant to antibiotics, resulting in a public health cost, as well. Yet, the standard approach of treating all pneumonia with antibiotics makes perfect sense. At the time of diagnosis, the specific germ responsible is unknown, so whether the pneumonia will respond to antibiotics is unknown. Withholding treatment of a pneumonia that turns out to be bacterial would increase the risk of developing worsening illness and complications, so the benefit to the one-third who will respond makes it well worth treating two-thirds unnecessarily.

At no cost at all, with widespread benefit from a better diet and estimating even just a few accruing benefit from prevention of food allergy, an Eat The Eight intervention makes equally good sense.

Comparison to Medication for a Mental Health Disorder

According to a report in *Time Magazine* in 2017, "Clinical depression affects about 16 million people in the U.S. and is estimated to cost about $210 billion a year in productivity loss and health care needs."

One of the most common and growing treatments for depression is a class of medications known as selective serotonin reuptake inhibitors (SSRI's). Early studies showed that SSRI's are very effective in alleviating the symptoms of severely affected and hospitalized patients. Hoping to provide benefit to more people, the use of these medications was expanded to patients with milder depression and other related conditions, such as anxiety. The results of subsequent studies, which were designed differently and included patients with milder depression, have concluded that SSRI's might not be much more effective than placebo (sugar pills).

Some experts believe that patients with milder depression derive less benefit than those with more severe depression, but still do derive some benefit from SSRI's. Whether, how much, and for whom SSRI's are beneficial remains controversial, as experts debate the results of studies. In the meantime, in the face of an enormous number of people with depression, the enormous societal burden of depression, the resultant demand for treatment, and the pressure this puts on the prescribers to do something (is this beginning to sound familiar?), millions of people continue to take SSRI's at a cost of billions of dollars annually. (I would be remiss if I didn't mention the contribution of the pharmaceutical industry—through advertising and sales calls to physicians' offices—to the growing use of these medications. After all, sales figures indicate that SSRIs have been a huge cash cow for the drug-makers.) In other words, *when the burden of illness is high, society is willing to spend billions of dollars for a treatment with questionable efficacy when it has been shown that there is potential for benefit.*

The same calculus would certainly lead to a recommendation for infants to Eat The Eight—at no cost.

Comparison to Antibiotics for Strep Throat

The previous examples, although by no means esoteric, are not so common as to be part of almost everyone's experience. Also, it seems safe to assume that the average person would not expect a simple and straightforward rationale behind the diagnosis and treatment of those conditions. Strep throat, on the other hand, with an estimated several million cases annually, is a condition that almost everyone has experienced first or second hand. It is also generally perceived to be simple to diagnose and treat as the result of how patients experience a visit for sore throat when they come to the office: the patient arrives in my office with a sore throat and possibly other symptoms such as fever and headache; my exam reveals a throat infection and no other apparent reason for the symptoms; and a swab of the throat is done to test for the presence of the strep germ. If the test shows strep (these days most office tests for strep are of the rapid variety, providing a result within minutes) I will write a prescription for an antibiotic, which the patient (or parent) understands is necessary to eradicate the infection in order to relieve their symptoms. The reality, however, is that the diagnosis is not as clear cut as the result of a rapid test. The reason to treat has almost nothing to do with eradicating infection of the throat, and necessity for treatment might itself be debatable.

It is no wonder that I see many children with sore throat every week, as it is the reason for 2-4% of visits to family practitioners, 2.8% of all Emergency Department visits for children 15 and under, and a total of about 11,000,000 annual visits to the doctor. About 20-25% of sore throats are caused by strep. One study estimated the cost of strep throat in children at $224 to $539 million annually.

Symptoms of strep throat typically include sore throat, fever, and headache, but severe complications can occur. These include peri-tonsillar abscess (collection of pus around the tonsils), which can often be treated with antibiotics but sometimes requires surgery to drain the abscess; and acute rheumatic fever (ARF), which occurs as a result of an autoimmune response to the initial infection. ARF can include inflammation of blood vessels, joints, the nervous system, and, of greatest concern, the heart (RHD—rheumatic heart disease). Fifty percent of patients with ARF will have RHD, which can result in significant damage to the heart's valves leading to significant compromise and even death. Having strep throat is uncomfortable, but, although generally not discussed at an office visit for sore throat, it is the potential complication of RHD that is by far of greatest concern.

In 1943, after an outbreak of strep throat at a military base in Wyoming resulted in many cases of ARF, a study showed that one case of ARF was prevented for every 50-60 trainees who were treated with antibiotics. Based on this, treating strep throat with antibiotics became routine medical practice—*but not to relieve the sore throat.* Prior to the advent of antibiotics, strep throat was treated like the common cold—"take two aspirin and call me in the morning"—and the infection *does resolve without antibiotics*. The purpose of the antibiotic is to prevent the complications of ARF and RHD, so treating strep throat would appear to be the obvious thing to do—except that these complications of strep throat, although still a significant problem in much of the developing world, have been decreasing in developed nations for 100 years, *the decline having started well before the use of antibiotics*. The precise reasons for this are unclear, but have been attributed to some combination of less overcrowding, better hygiene, and changes in the strep germ itself, among other factors. To be clear, antibiotics have also contributed to the decline of ARF and RHD, but how much of the decline can be attributed specifically to the use of antibiotics is unknown.

A comprehensive review of our approach to strep throat published in 1985 noted that although we do not have adequate information about the possible cofactors involved in contracting ARF or RHD, from the clinical point of view "*the low risk of rheumatic fever today suggests that perhaps we should reassess present policies regarding our hunt for the* streptococcus *and our determination to eradicate it*" (italics mine). It's not that the evidence isn't solid that antibiotics treat strep and prevent some cases of ARF and RHD. Rather, the question is "are the benefits of treating strep throat with antibiotics greater than the costs?"

A review of the data in 2015 calculated the utility of treating strep throat with antibiotics, with the understanding that the reason for treatment is to prevent ARF that could lead to RHD. Given the rarity of ARF and RHD, the authors concluded that the number needed to treat (NNT) to prevent one case of ARF is 10,000; to prevent one case of RHD, 20,000; and to prevent one death from RHD 5,000,000. Is this too much treatment for too little prevention? That depends on the cost of treatment. Apart from the expense of all those visits, strep tests, and antibiotics, for every 5,000,000 children treated with antibiotics, it is estimated that "12,500 will experience anaphylaxis [to the antibiotic] and 137 can be expected to die of their anaphylactic reaction." This clearly suggests that the cost of treatment may outweigh the benefit.

It is known that strep sore throat is most common in children 5 to 15 years of age in the winter and spring months. If we tested and treated only this group during those months, the NNT would be more favorable. With this in mind, guidelines from the Infectious Diseases Society of America recommend strep throat not be tested for in children less than three years of age who appear to have a virus, due to the extremely low risk of ARF. Despite this, physicians and parents alike generally fear much more the potential negative consequences of not treating a condition rather than the risks associated with treatment, so this guideline is not strictly followed. "Appears to have a virus" is not quite the same as "I'm sure it's a virus;" parental pressure to do a strep test on every sore throat cannot be overstated and clinicians have substantial and justifiable fear of under-diagnosing and undertreating.

Even if antibiotics are not necessary to prevent rheumatic fever, isn't it just a good idea to treat strep to cure the throat infection? As a matter of fact, although strep throat symptoms resolve about 16 hours more quickly when treated with antibiotics, if left untreated strep throat infection will resolve on its own.

What about preventing peri-tonsillar abscess? Although it is possible that some cases could be prevented, it is likely that very few would be, because peri-tonsillar abscess is generally already present when the patient is first seen and there is little evidence that treating strep throat prevents them.

To further complicate matters, it is known that approximately 10% of children carry strep bacteria in their throat. If a throat culture is done on a strep carrier, they will test positive and be treated; but they are not infected, are not at increased risk of infection, do not put those around them at risk, and do not need treatment. Determining that a child with a sore throat and positive throat culture is a carrier rather than infected with strep requires a blood test that is neither practical to obtain nor easily interpreted. So approximately 10% of children treated with antibiotics for a positive strep test are exposed to the risks of treatment with no possibility of benefit.

In the final analysis, it is no surprise that one reviewer concluded, "*any relaxation of our currently recommended approaches to streptococcal infections should be undertaken with great caution,* since we do not understand the reasons for the decline and consequently cannot fully anticipate the possible results of any relaxation in policy." Consistent with this, an overview of rheumatic fever from the well-known and highly regarded Mayo Clinic states, "Rheumatic fever is an inflammatory disease that can develop as a complication of inadequately treated strep throat or scarlet fever [rash and fever associated with strep throat]. The only way to prevent rheumatic fever is to treat strep throat infections or scarlet fever promptly with a full course of appropriate antibiotics."

There can be little doubt that strep throat does cause RF, but the evidence appears to show that *it does not cause RF on its own.* It is multifactorial, meaning that strep throat might result in RF in the presence of other factors such as genetic predisposition, a specific strep throat germ type (as opposed to all strep throat germs), and/or other health and hygiene issues. In the absence of certain knowledge about these factors in any individual case of strep throat, the standard is to simply treat all strep throats.

When unable to determine precisely which individual patient with symptoms actually needs intervention, medical teaching contends that it is sometimes not only acceptable *but also necessary to treat some who do not need treatment in order to be sure none who do need treatment are missed,* even if the treatment is quite invasive. I was taught a classic example of this during my surgical rotation in medical school when a senior surgeon explained that because the diagnosis of appendicitis was impossible to make with certainty based on a physical exam and labs (that were available at that time), if 15% of the patients he operated on for appendicitis were not found to have a normal appendix, he was doing too few appendectomies and was certain to send home a patient with appendicitis. There was broad consensus about this in the medical community based on the risks and benefits of doing the surgery and the risks of sending home a patient with appendicitis. (To be clear, with vastly improved imaging modalities—CT, MRI, Ultrasound—the diagnosis of appendicitis is far more precise and the number of patients taken to the operating room unnecessarily is much smaller. This example is classic, but outdated—no surgeon today would make the same assertion my attending did over 30 years ago.)

It is evident that in the setting of uncertain evidence, when the balance of risk and benefit of treatment is ambiguous or unsettled, and the potential outcome of not treating is a rare but significant disease, the consensus of medical opinion is to persist in prescribing treatment that for many is almost certainly unnecessary. By the same reasoning, it should be far easier to come to a consensus that infants ought to Eat The Eight. If early introduction should somehow turn out to be ineffective as allergy prevention for some or even many, they would still benefit from the improved diet and have not been subjected to any risk from the intervention.

Describing how medical advice and treatments are sometimes supported by a delicate foundation feels a little like pulling the curtain back on the Wizard of Oz. However, the point is not to suggest that current advice or treatments are inappropriate or make the general public uneasy, but rather to understand the context of medical advice in general. In "What Doctors Don't Know (Almost Everything)," *New York Times*, 2002, Dr. Kevin Patterson states, "The vast majority of medical therapies, it is now clear, have never been evaluated by systematic study [...]" (I recommend you read this *New York Times* article in its entirety, it is eye opening and wonderfully written.) A review on the strength of scientific evidence cited work from the 1970s that '"more than half of all medical treatments, and perhaps as many as 85 percent, have never been validated by clinical trials.'" Although this has improved somewhat over time, it remains largely true due to the lack of the resources necessary to produce evidence that would provide strong support for medical recommendations.

Studies like LEAP are exceptional because they require sufficient funding, expertise, a lot of work, and some luck to do well. That LEAP so well overcame these barriers and produced statistically impressive results explains its lofty standing. (It is difficult to overstate the import of LEAP. In the last eight years, 281,304 clinical studies have been registered. In 2016, the Society for Clinical Trials presented LEAP with the 2015 Trial of the Year Award.) It also means that additional strong evidence for early introduction of the Big Eight foods is not something we can reasonably expect any time soon (although some additional studies are underway).

I have already shown that a recommendation to Eat The Eight is strongly supported on the basis of the evidence and cost-benefit analysis. It is now also clear that the strength of this support surpasses accepted medical standards.

CHAPTER IX

If You Could Prevent Food Allergy with Real Food, Why Use a Substitute?

"Let thy food be thy medicine, and let thy medicine be thy food."

(Hippocrates, Father of Medicine)

"Ain't nothin' like the real thing baby, ain't nothin' like the real thing."

(Ashford and Simpson)

ONE OF THE THINGS I love about early introduction of the Big Eight is that the intervention requires nothing more than feeding nutritious foods to infants. Make no mistake, I have seen and administered some miraculous new treatments over the last 30 years and I do deeply appreciate that they are available. For example, I am reminded every time I see an infant get the Hib vaccine (which was introduced as I neared the end of my residency in pediatrics) that I have not seen in years the life-threatening infections the Hib bacteria can cause and that I did see all too often during my training. Also, during my residency I saw some of the first children treated for HIV/AIDS, which at that time, due to mostly ineffective treatments, yielded nothing but frustration and sadness. Today, thanks to the treatment now available, I have a teenage patient who was born with HIV and has been healthy her entire life. Vaccines and medications can do miraculous good, but are never without some amount of risk and expense—there is no free lunch.

Fortunately, there is an exception to every rule and with Eat The Eight lunch *is* free—because *Eat The Eight is lunch.* No one can guarantee that an infant won't react to these foods. On the contrary, some certainly will. But with no risk of side effect, an infant's risk of developing food allergy can be reduced while they benefit additionally from a more nutritious diet, *just by eating these foods.*

Despite this, products have been developed to medicalize early introduction of The Big Eight, substituting powders or liquid derived from food as an alternative to actual food.

SimplyPeanut

On February 20, 2017, a press release announced the availability of SimplyPeanut, a product created to introduce peanut to infants, with the claim, "Peanut Introduction for Infants is Now Simple and Safe." SimplyPeanut is peanut protein flour in pre-measured packets, each providing one gram of peanut protein. It is recommended that infants consume two packets daily, three times a week. (The LEAP study proved that about two grams of peanut protein about three times a week prevented peanut allergy; this amount of peanut protein was chosen for the study based on the approximate average intake of peanut protein by infants in Israel, which was the inspiration for LEAP. It seems sensible to recommend this amount of intake—about two grams, about three times a week—as a general goal.) Vitamins have been added to the peanut flour with the claim that this makes it "the ideal immune boost product for your infant." The cost is $25 for a one-month supply. While it is true that this product ought to provide infants the same peanut allergy prevention benefit as actual food, it is not clear why vitamins need to be added or how they provide an "immune boost," why one would choose it over real food, or what would justify the expense.

SimplyPeanut is simple and safe, but the LEAP study already showed us that *introducing real peanut food to infants is simple and safe.*

"Hello, Peanut!"

A month later, "Hello, Peanut!" was launched as the "first and only product available for parents to safely introduce peanuts to infants," although it was demonstrably neither first nor only. Made of sprouted oat flakes and peanut powder, the product is packaged as a "gradual system for peanut introduction." Feedings are started with the

Introduction Kit, which contains seven packets of product with gradually increasing amounts of peanut protein for the first seven days. Feedings are then continued with the Maintenance Kit, each packet containing a constant amount of peanut protein. This system is based on how allergists perform oral food challenges to diagnose food allergy, starting with small amounts of the food at first and then gradually increasing that amount, until there is a reaction or it is determined that the patient is not allergic. Although this approach is safe, LEAP showed that there is no need to introduce peanut in this more complicated manner. Again, this product offers no additional benefit over simply eating food.

The introductory kit costs $25 and covers the first week. The maintenance kit is $20 and contains eight packets. It is recommended that infants consume one to three packets a week, which would result in a peanut protein intake of one to three grams a week. This is not unreasonable, but it is arbitrary. When recommending early introduction of the Big Eight foods, most would suggest simply an intake of "early and often." Hello, Peanut! recommends continued use of their product until infants can eat whole peanuts or peanut butter. This would result in at least a four-year commitment to the product, as undiluted peanut butter is generally not recommended before four years of age and peanuts not before five years of age in order to avoid the risk of choking. It also disregards the broadly accepted advice that peanut food can be safely fed to infants in the safe forms of diluted peanut butter and peanut puff snacks. The safety of feeding real peanut food to infants is borne out by a long track record in Israel and the LEAP study.

Aralyte

The same month that "Hello, Peanut!" was introduced as "the first and only," Antera Therapeutics launched Aralyte, the third "first and only commercial product based on LEAP for early peanut introduction." Unlike the others, Aralyte was a liquid form of peanut protein packaged in a vial. The company described their product as "an all-natural, organic food for special dietary use that offers parents a safe and structured means of implementing the LEAP regimen." Like the others, Aralyte was not a food; in seeking a safer, more structured way of feeding peanut to infants, it, too, filled a need that doesn't exist. As an added measure of "safety," it was intended that the system be initiated in the physician's office and then prescribed for home use. Because it was so expensive—one could accomplish with $2 worth of peanut butter what would require $180 dollars-worth of product—and satisfied no apparent need, Aralyte was the subject of much criticism. (For the complete story, see David Zweig's excellent article in *The Verge*, "Antera Therapeutics Announces First and Only Commercial Product Based on LEAP for Early Peanut Introduction.") It appears that the product no longer exists, as I have been unable to find it online.

SpoonfulONE

The company Before Brands has gone beyond peanut with SpoonfulONE, a product that is made of "a powder blend of gentle servings" (I do not know what a gentle serving is) of less than one gram total of "peanuts, milk, eggs, almonds, soy, wheat, shrimp, cashews, hazelnuts, oat, cod, pecans, salmon, sesame, walnuts, and pistachios." They recommend that infants and children consume one packet daily and that this be continued as the child grows, even after the child begins to consume the included foods. A one-month supply is $69.90, discounted to $59.50 with a subscription.

While I applaud the Eat The Eight concept, there is universal agreement among pediatricians and allergists that new foods be introduced to infants one at a time, with not more than one new food introduced every few days, thereby making it easier to identify the cause of an allergic reaction should there be one. It is surprising that the Before Brands' pediatricians and allergists created a product that exposes infants to all of these allergens at the same time. In addition to that, there is no data to support the arbitrary protein dose in the packet, there's no way to know until what age to continue, and given the real food alternative, there is no justification for the expense. As Marina Chaparro, a clinical dietitian and national spokesperson for the Academy of Nutrition and Dietetics put it, "It really misses the mark in terms of teaching kids how to start learning how to eat. With food solids, you're exposing that child to not just the nutrients, but we're also teaching children how to like that food, learning how to adjust to different textures, and how to have that bite of whole wheat bread." She recommends instead that parents "invest in an array of various foods and educate themselves on how to properly introduce them into a baby's diet."

In other words, Eat The *Real Food* Eight.

CHAPTER X

Eczema and Early Introduction

"Beauty is being comfortable and confident in your own

skin."

(Iman, Fashion Model)

ECZEMA AND EXPOSURE TO ALLERGENS are important factors very closely related to the concept of early introduction of the Big Eight. Understanding this relationship can further explain why early introduction is so important and also point to additional interventions that would be safe and sensible to reduce an infant's risk of developing food allergy.

Exposure to peanut through inflamed skin was identified as a risk factor for peanut allergy in March of 2003. A study by Dr. Gideon Lack noted that up until that time the only known risk factors for developing peanut allergy were a family history of peanut allergy and the presence of atopic (allergic) disease. It was known that foods could make eczema worse and a previous study had even suggested that peanut allergy could cause eczema. Dr. Lack's study showed that there was a relationship between the use of skin preparations that contained peanut oil (in products used to treat eczema) and peanut allergy, indicating that perhaps it was the other way around with *eczema leading to peanut allergy*. It was suggested that besides peanut oil, peanut butter could potentially cause sensitization by exposure through the skin before an infant has eaten peanut. If this were so, ongoing exposure through the skin might also explain why peanut allergy is generally not outgrown.

How likely is it that an infant could come into contact with peanut in the environment prior to actually eating peanut? It turns out that it is extremely likely. Fully 90% of US households report eating peanut butter and it had been observed that there was a relationship between peanut consumption in the home and peanut allergy. A study done in September 2013 showed that in households where peanut is eaten, peanut protein will be found in the dust around an infant's bed, crib rail, and play area.

Previous studies had already shown that individuals with eczema do not have adequate protection against environmental (not food) allergens due to a defective skin barrier. In July 2013, a study that used data from the ongoing EAT study showed that infants with eczema are over six times more likely than infants without eczema to be sensitized (having developed defensive proteins called antibodies in response to an allergen) to a variety of foods including egg, cow's milk, and peanut. These infants had not yet eaten any solid foods, suggesting that the sensitization occurred through the skin. The researchers concluded that although sensitization does not always lead to actual symptoms of allergy, these findings suggested that if the eczema is adequately treated, it might also reduce the risk of food allergies.

The studies showing that infants are sensitized to food through the skin, along with the LEAP study showing that early feeding of peanut to high-risk infants prevents peanut allergy, together provide strong evidence that *when an infant is first (and continuously) exposed to food through eating, allergy is unlikely.* When early exposure occurs through the skin, the risk of allergy is increased.

Food can indeed cause eczema, but rather than eliminate an allergenic food from the diet of an infant with eczema but no actual evidence of specific allergy to that food (as is sometimes done), the correct approach is to *Eat The Eight and repair the skin barrier by treating the eczema very aggressively.* If there is reason to suspect an infant has had an allergic reaction to a food and in order to treat eczema appropriately, it is important to have the guidance of a pediatric provider and possibly an allergist as well.

Given the current information, the best strategy to prevent food allergy in infants with eczema is to minimize exposure to allergens through the skin and maximize exposure through eating. So, Eat The Eight, but be sure also to *soothe the skin.*

CHAPTER XI

How to Eat The Eight

"First, introducing such an allergenic food to an at risk baby

of only 4 to 6 months is intimidating to contemplate, and

the polar opposite of the avoidance messages we have

etched into our brains. And second, the whole 'when to

introduce foods question' has now, officially, been turned on

its head. That, my friends, is a lot to absorb."

(Gwen Smith in "Food Allergy, a LEAP into an Allergic Culture Change," March 15, 2016.)

THE LEAP STUDY, ALONG WITH the other studies and opinions that support a recommendation of early introduction of the Big Eight, filled me with an enthusiastic sense of opportunity to help decrease infants' risk of developing food allergy. I believed that parents would embrace these guidelines, but before very long it was clear that they had not done so.

When I asked Eran, a friend in Israel, if he and his wife had experienced anxiety before introducing peanut or any other food to his children when they were infants, he was confused. After a brief lesson on the topic of food allergy and infant feeding in the US, he responded emphatically, "Of course not!" In a country where the introduction of peanut has never been delayed intentionally, starting an infant on new foods is not a stressful experience.

In countries where parents have delayed the introduction of the Big Eight foods, on the other hand, the proponents of early introduction—myself included, after my experience while doing research for this book—understand that it's not quite so simple.

—It can be difficult to let go of old beliefs:

"The early guidelines were the ones that took hold and that's still what a lot of primary care providers, as well as families, are believing to be true. We have a lot of years of misconceptions to undo here, so that's part of the problem." (Dr. David Stukus, Associate Professor of Pediatrics, Section of Allergy and Immunology at Nationwide Children's Hospital, noted at the ACAAI meeting in Boston October 2017.)

—Making parenting decisions is not always easy:

"EAT reinforces how complex and difficult it is to be a parent, and to try to feed your child and do the right thing. When you get these negative perceptions of foods [as a result of the old advice], it puts a lot of stress on families. I think the good news about this information is that *there's no reason not to do this, there's no harm that has come from early introduction."* (James Baker, FARE; italics mine.)

—It is easy to forget that early introduction is about good nutrition:

"Food allergens are healthy foods, things like cow's milk, peanuts, tree nuts, sesame. If you aren't allergic, you want to be eating them in a balanced diet." (Dr. George Du Toit, LEAP investigator.) (Sesame is not one of the Big Eight. Although the exact prevalence of sesame allergy is unknown, there have been reports that it has been increasing. Concern that it is a major allergen has led FARE and others to advocate that the Food Allergen Labeling and Consumer Protection Act (FALCPA) be expanded to include sesame as a major allergen. Nosh The Nine?)

—Change is sometimes easier one step at a time:

"We don't need to achieve perfection, but we do need to make progress." (Dr. David Stukus.)

When ready for early introduction of the Big Eight, how should a parent proceed?

First, parents should know that none of the recent findings about the early introduction of foods for infants has changed certain basic sound advice we have been giving for years: start solids when an infant is developmentally ready—usually between four and six months of age—and introduce only one new food every few days. (Note: the AAP recommends exclusive breast feeding for the first six months. Developmental readiness is demonstrated by having good head control while seated in a high chair; displaying interest in foods by, for example, reaching for them; and then swallowing, rather than rejecting, a small amount of food placed in the mouth. As always, parents should discuss the introduction of solids with their pediatric provider.)

To avoid any misconception about the idea that *absolutely any food* is OK when solids are started, it is important to remember that honey still should not be introduced prior to one year of age. This is not due to the risk of allergic reaction, but rather the risk of botulism. (Honey can be contaminated with botulism spores that produce a toxin that causes muscle weakness or paralysis. Infants under 12 months are at risk for this because, unlike older children and adults, the spores produce the toxin only in an immature digestive tract. Despite the importance of avoiding honey, it is reassuring to note that the risk is greatest to infants less than six months of age, prior to which many have not eaten any solids; only a small percentage of honey contains botulism spores; and with proper treatment, the vast majority of affected infants recover completely.)

Most experts recommend starting the Big Eight after having started a few other foods. There seems to be no particularly compelling reason to do this, other than establishing that the infant is ready for solids and possibly to help make a parent feel more comfortable introducing foods that they previously believed their infant shouldn't eat.

One good guide for how to introduce particular foods is, again, Dr. Tanya Altmann's *What to Feed Your Baby*, with tips on introducing fish, egg, dairy, and nuts.

Regarding dairy, it is important to understand that infants, whether breastfed or taking formula, should not have milk prior to age one. In terms of early introduction, milk really means foods made from milk, like yogurt and cheese.

Avoidance of foods an infant could choke on is perhaps the most important principle to follow when starting solids. Among the Big Eight foods, this applies most obviously to peanut and tree nuts. As noted previously, when baby is developmentally ready, peanut can be introduced as peanut butter puffs such as Puffworks baby, peanut butter diluted with water or other soft food, or peanut flour added to other soft food.

I would be remiss as a pediatrician if I didn't mention that breastfeeding, both prior to starting solids and after solids have been introduced, may decrease the risk of developing allergy to food. UpToDate, an authoritative, evidence-based, clinical decision support service for medical providers notes, "Exclusive breastfeeding in the first four months of life may decrease the risk of cow's milk allergy in early childhood." Studies have also shown that breastfeeding can reduce the risk of developing eczema, which might subsequently reduce the risk of developing food allergy (see Chapter IX), although the evidence for this has been mixed. Results of a study published in 2017 suggest that the most effective way to reduce sensitization to peanut is for a mother to eat peanut *and* breast feed *and* introduce peanut to baby in the first year of life. Going even a bit further back in the relationship between mother and infant, a study from 2014 found a lower incidence of peanut and tree nut allergy in the infants of mothers who ate peanut and tree nut during pregnancy. These studies do not prove with absolute certainty that maternal consumption of peanut during pregnancy and/or breast feeding prevents infants from developing allergy. They do, however, make it clear that pregnant and breast feeding mothers not only need not avoid these foods, but, just as with infants, can and should eat these foods for their nutritional value and the reasonable likelihood that doing so contributes to decreased food allergy risk for their infants.

When, how much, and how often do infants need to Eat The Eight? The simple answer is early and often.

LEAP study infants began peanut between four and less than 11 months of age. The EAT study enrolled infants as young as three months. It is possible that feeding the Big Eight prior to the usually recommended four to six months of age for starting solids is safe and beneficial, but there is too little evidence to recommend that. On the other end of the spectrum, although the Big Eight foods have nutritional benefit at any age after four months, experts believe that the window for early introduction to prevent food allergy closes by 11 months. Again, four to six months seems to make the most sense.

The LEAP study infants were fed approximately two grams of peanut protein approximately three times weekly and the results showed this to be effective in preventing peanut allergy. This does not, however, prove that this is the exact right amount.

The EAT study protocol set an intentionally high target of three grams of protein of five or more foods per week for five or more weeks, with the understanding that the specific amount of food that needs to be eaten to prevent allergy is unknown. If this feels challenging, the EAT study experience reveals that it certainly can be, as many parents failed to follow the protocol stringently. On the other hand, the study also revealed that despite the fear of an allergic reaction, parents were willing to introduce allergenic foods including peanut into their infant's diet at less than six months of age. Also, although many families failed to follow the protocol to the letter, most infants did at least try most of the foods.

Another study pointed out that partial adherence to early introduction did not lead to food allergy. In other words, there was no harm in trying.

For how long must infants and children Eat The Eight in order to avoid developing food allergy? In the LEAP study, children were fed peanut until age five years and, again, this proved to be effective. Still, we do not know precisely how long an infant needs to eat allergenic foods to achieve tolerance.

LEAP-ON, a follow-up study to LEAP, showed that infants who ate peanut early and then stopped eating peanut for one year remained free of peanut allergy. Again, no one can say with certainty for how long an infant can stop eating peanut and remain allergy-free, but as Dr. Gerald Nepom, Director of the Immune Tolerance Network put it, "This study offers reassurance that eating peanut-containing foods as part of a normal diet—with occasional periods of time without peanut—will be a safe practice for most children following successful tolerance therapy [early introduction]." It is important to remember that *the Big Eight foods are not a treatment, they are good nutrition.*

Some years ago I had the good fortune to see Michael Pollan talk about his then new book, *In Defense of Food.* He joked that when his editor added the subtitle "Eat Food. Not Too Much. Mostly Plants," it was no longer necessary to read the rest of the book. With that in mind, I have saved my EBM-inspired summary for the end of this book:

—The Big Eight foods can safely be added to the diet of infants; the evidence for this is extremely strong.

—The early introduction of the Big Eight foods is very likely to decrease an infant's risk of developing allergy to these foods; the evidence for this is rapidly developing.

—Adding the Big Eight foods to an infant's diet will improve their nutrition; the evidence for this is incontrovertible.

With this information, a parent can now decide how to proceed.

Perhaps you would really just prefer to know what I would do with my own children? That's easy--I would have them

Eat The Eight, early and often ...

Eat The Eight, early and often ...

Eat The Eight, early and often ...

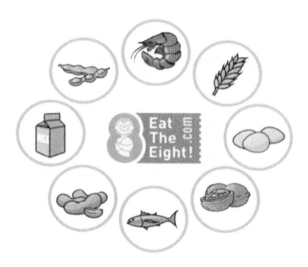

Notes on Sources

Chapter I

Lau GY, "Anxiety and Stress in Mothers of Food-allergic Children," *Pediatric Allergy and Immunology*, 2014 May;25(3):236-42.

"A Growing Food Allergy Epidemic: One in 13 U.S. Children Has a Food Allergy," KidsWithFoodAllergies.org, 5/13/15.

"Food Allergy Facts and Statistics for the U.S.," Food Allergy & Education, foodallergy.org.

Miller, D., "Current and Emerging Immunotherapeutic Approaches to Treat and Prevent Peanut Allergy," *Expert Review of Vaccines*, 2012:11 (12):1471-1481.

Macdougall, CF, at al., "How Dangerous is Food Allergy in Childhood? The Incidence of Severe and Fatal Allergic Reactions Across UK and Ireland," *Archives of Disease in Childhood*, 2002; 86: 236-239.

Mayer, C., et al., "Does Currently Available Data Support the Use of Oral Immunotherapy Treatments," *Infectious Diseases in Children*, May 2018, healio.com.

Turner, P., MD, "Fatal Anaphylaxis: Mortality Rate and Risk Factors," *Journal of Allergy and Clinical Immunology Practice*, 2017 Sep-Oct; 5(5): 1169–1178.

Gupta, R., et al., "The Economic Impact of Childhood Food Allergy in the United States," *Journal of the American Medical Association Pediatrics*, 2013 Nov; 167 (11):1026-31.

Tran, M, et. al., "Predicting the Atopic March: Results from the Canadian Healthy Infant Longitudinal Development Study," *Journal of Allergy and Clinical Immunolgy*, February 2018 Volume 141, Issue 2, Pages 601–607 e8.

Watson, W., MD, Professor and Associate Chair, Department of Pediatrics, Dalhousie University, "The Burden of Food Allergy," Grand Rounds presentation at British Columbia Children's Hospital on January 10, 2014.

Smith, G., "Sabrina's Law Turns 10 Years Old," *Allergic Living*, May 5, 2015.

Dean, J., "Disclosing Food Allergy Status in Schools: Health-related Stigma Among School Children in Ontario," *Health and Social Care in the Community*, March 19, 2015.

Sicherer, S., MD, et al., "The Impact of Childhood Food Allergy on Quality of Life," *Annals of Allergy, Asthma, and Immunology*, December 2001, Volume 87, Issue 6, pages 461–464.

Boesveld, S., "Oh, The Humanities!: Food Allergies Can Mean Loneliness, Social Isolation for Children: Researcher," *National Post*, May 31, 2012.

Chapter II

"Food Allergies, A Growing Health Concern," FAIR health, fairhealth.org.

Waggoner, M., "Parsing the Peanut Panic: The Social Life of a Contested Food Allergy Epidemic," *Social Sciences and Medicine*, 2013 Aug; 90: 49–55. Published online, 2013 May 6.

Sampson, H., "Food Allergy: Past, Present and Future," *Allergology International* 65, October 2016, October;65(4):363-369.

Hopkins, J., "The Very Intolerant Peanut," *Food and Chemical Toxicology*, Vol. 33, No. 1, pp 81-86, 1995.

Assem, ES, et al., "Anaphylaxis Induced by Peanuts," *British Medical Journal*, 1990; 300:1377-8.

Donovan, K., et al., "Vegetable Burger Allergy: All Was Nut As It Appeared," *British Medical Journal*, 1990; 300: 1378.

Smith, T., "Allergy to Peanuts", *British Medical Journal*, Vol. 300, May 26, 1990; 300:1354.

McSharry, C., "Allergy to Peanuts," *British Medical Journal*, Vol. 300, 1990 Jun 30; 300(6741):1726.

Ackroyd, JF, "Allergy to Peanuts" *British Medical Journal*, Vol. 301, 1990 Jul 14; 301(6743):120.

Zeiger, R., "The Development and Prediction of Atopy in High-risk Children: Follow-Up at Age Seven Years in a Prospective Randomized Study of Combined Maternal and Infant Food Allergen Avoidance," *Journal of Allergy Clinical Immunology*, 1995, Jun;95(6):1179-90.

"Hypoallergenic Infant Formulas," Committee on Nutrition, *Pediatrics* 2000;106;346.

Claridge, J., et al., "History and Development of Evidence-based Medicine," *World Journal of Surgery*, 2005 May;29(5):547-53.

Sur, R., et al., "History of Evidence-based Medicine," *Indian Journal of Urology*, 2011 Oct-Dec; 27(4): 487–489.

Lohr, K., "Rating the Strength of Scientific Evidence: Relevance for Quality Improvement Programs," *International Journal for Quality in Health Care*, Vol. 16, Issue 1, February 1, 2004:9-18.

Ebell, M., et al., "Strength of Recommendation Taxonomy (SORT): A Patient- Centered Approach to Grading Evidence in the Medical Literature," *American Family Physician*, 2004 February 1;69(3):548-556.

Patterson, K., "What Drs. Don't Know (Almost Everything), *New York Times Magazine*, May 5, 2002.

Barraclough, K., "Why Doctors Don't Read Research Papers," *British Medical Journal,* December 11, 2004;329:1411.

Jiwa, M., "Doctors and Medical Science," *Australasian Medical Journal,* 9/9/2012;5(8): 462-467.

Gabbay, J. et al., "Evidence Based Guidelines or Collectively Constructed 'Mindlines?' Ethnographic Study of Knowledge Management in Primary Care," *British Medical Journal,* 2004 October 30; 329(7473):1013.

Oransky, I., et al.,"Two Cheers for the Retraction Boom," *The New Atlantis,* Spring/Summer 2016.

O'Donnell, M., "Why Doctors Don't Read Research Papers; Scientific Papers Are Not Written to Disseminate Information," *British Medical Journal,* 2005 Jan 29;330(7485):256.

Loadsman, J., "Widening the Search for Suspect Data – Is the Flood of Retractions About to Become a Tsunami?" *Anaesthesia,* 2017 August;72(8):931-935.

Kolbert, E., "Why Facts Don't Change Our Minds," *New Yorker,* February 27, 2017.

"Food Allergy Facts and Statistics for the U.S.," Food Allergy Research & Education, foodallergyorg.com.

Chapter III

Greer, FR, et al. and the Committee on Nutrition and Section on Allergy and Immunology, "Effects of Early Nutritional Interventions on the Development of Atopic Disease in Infants and Children: The Role of Maternal Dietary Restriction, Breastfeeding, Timing of Introduction of Complementary Foods, and Hydrolyzed Formulas," *Pediatrics*, 2008 Jan;121(1):183-91.

Louden, K., "New Guidelines Downplay Role of Diet in Preventing Pediatric Allergies: An Expert Interview With Frank Greer, MD," *Medscape*, Apr. 21, 2008.

Lehman, S., "Doctors May Not Follow Peanut Guidelines for Allergy-Prone Babies," *Health News*, August 29, 2018.

Bilton, N., "The American Diet: 34 Gigabytes a Day," *New York Times*, December 9, 2009.

Jiwa, M., "Doctors and Medical Science," *Australasian Medical Journal*, 9/9/2012; 5(8): 462-467.

Kolbert, E., "Why Facts Don't Change Our Minds," *The New Yorker*, Feb. 27, 2017.

Scanlan, M., "Why Does Nutrition Advice Constantly Change?", *The Nutrition Press*, March 22, 2018.

Ioannidis, J., "The Challenge of Reforming Nutritional Epidemiologic Research," *Journal of the American Medical Association*, 2018;320(10):969-970.

Kharasch, E., "Errors and Integrity in Seeking and Reporting Apparent Research Misconduct," *Anesthesiology*, 2017 Nov;127(5):733-737.

Oransky, I., "Two Cheers for the Retraction Boom," *The New Atlantis*, Spring/Summer 2016.

Rabin, R., "Major Study of Drinking Will Be Shut Down," *New York Times*, June 15, 2018.

Rabin, R., "Anheuser-Busch to Pull Funding From Major Alcohol Study," *New York Times*, June 8, 2018.

Ornstein, C., et al., "Top Cancer Researcher Fails to Disclose Corporate Financial Ties in Major Research Journals," *New York Times*, Sept. 8, 2018.

Sherman, S., "The Psychology of Collective Responsibility: When and Why Collective Entities Are Likely To Be Held Responsible For the Misdeeds of Individual Members," *Journal of Law and Policy*, Vol. 19, Issue 1, 2010; 137-170.

Thomson, J., "Can One Bad Apple Really Spoil A Whole Barrel? We Found Out," *Huffington Post*, July 13, 2016.

"Do Vaccines Cause Autism," *The History of Vaccines*, The College of Physicians of Philadelphia.

Thompson, G., "Measles and MMR Statistics," *House of Commons Library*, October 2, 2009.

Gerber, J., "Vaccines and Autism: A Tale of Shifting Hypotheses," *Clinical Infectious Diseases*, Volume 48, Issue 4, 15 February 2009, Pages 456-461.

"Thimerosal in Vaccines", Centers for Disease Control and Prevention, cdc.gov.

Bulman, M., "Measles Eradicated in U.K. in 'Sign of Recovery' After MMR Vaccine Controversy," *Independent*, October 27, 2017.

"Many Americans Say Infectious and Emerging Diseases in Other Countries Will Threaten U.S.," ASM Communications, *American Society for Microbiology*, , May 21, 2018.

Olive, J., et al., "The State of the Antivaccine Movement in the United States: A Focused Examination of Nonmedical Exemptions in States and Counties," *PLOS Medicine*, June 12, 2018.

Bortz, K., "Nonmedical Vaccine Exemptions Increasing in US Metropolitan Areas," *Healio*, June 12, 2018. healio.com.

"Key Moments in Safe to Sleep® History: 1994-2003" at NIH.gov

Boyce, J., MD, et al., "Guidelines for the Diagnosis and Management of Food Allergy in the United States," Report of the NIAID-Sponsored Expert Panel, *Journal of Allergy and Clinical Immunology*, 2010 Dec; 126 (60):S1-58.

Chapter IV

Lack, G., "Epidemiologic Risks for Food Allergy", *Journal of Allergy and Clinical Immunology*, June 2008; 121(6):1331-6.

Lack, G., et al., "Early Consumption of Peanuts in Infancy is Associated with a Low Prevalence of Peanut Allergy," *Journal of Allergy Clinical. Immunology*, 2008 Nov.; 122(5):98491.

Du Toit, G., et al., "Identifying Infants at High Risk of Peanut Allergy: The Learning Early About Peanut Allergy (LEAP) Screening Study," *Journal of Allergy and Clinical Immunology*, January 2013;131(1):135-43.e1-12.

Du Toit, G., et al., "Randomized Trial of Peanut Consumption in Infants at Risk for Peanut Allergy," *New England Journal of Medicine*, Feb. 26, 2015, 2015; 372:803-813.

Poole, JA, et al., "Timing of Initial Exposure to Cereal Grains and the Risk of Wheat Allergy," *Pediatrics*, 2006 Jun;117(6):2175-82.

Prescott, SL, et al., "The Importance of Early Complementary Feeding in the Development of Oral Tolerance: Concerns and Controversies," *Pediatric Allergy and Immunology*, Aug 2008;19(5):375-80.

Wennergan, G., MD, PhD, "What If It is the Other Way Around? Early Introduction of Peanut and Fish Seems to Be Better Than Avoidance", *Acta Pediatrica*, 2009 Jul;98(7):1085-7.

Fleischer, DM, et al; Adverse Reaction to Foods Committee Report, "Primary Prevention of Allergic Disease Through Nutritional Interventions: Guidelines for Healthcare Professionals"; *Journal of Allergy and Clinical Immunology: In Practice* 2013;1:29-36.

Chan, E., et al., "Dietary Exposures and Allergy Prevention in High-risk Infants," *Paediatric Child Health*, 2013 Dec; 18(10): 545–549.

Sax, C., MD, "What Are the Healthiest Options for My Baby's First Solid Foods," Boston Children's Hospital Pediatric Health Blog, March 2014.

Green, T., MD, "Feeding Allergenic Foods to Babies and Pregnant or Nursing Moms," *Kids With Food Allergies*, website, April 2014.

The Anaphylaxis Campaign, PO Box 275, Farnborough, Hampshire GU14 6SX. Registered charity: 1085527, Press Release 2/24/15.

"Global Baby Puffs and Snacks Market - Drivers and Forecast from Technavio," *Business Wire*, online, February 9, 2017.

"Extruded Snacks: Puffing Up Sales," *Candy & Snack Today*, online, July 11, 2016.

Chapter V

"Consensus Communication on Early Peanut Introduction and the Prevention of Peanut Allergy in High-risk Infants," *Pediatrics*, September 2015, Vol. 136/Issue 3.

"Landmark Study Presented at AAAAI Annual Meeting Paves Way for Food Allergy Prevention," *Cision PRWeb*, online, February 23.2015.

Abrams, E., et al., "Food Introduction and Allergy Prevention in Infants," *Canadian Medical Association Journal*, November 17, 2015, 187 (17) 1297-1301.

"EAT Study: Early Introduction of Allergenic Foods to Induce Tolerance," *Food Standards Agency*, online, food.gov.uk.

Perkin, M., et al., "Randomized Trial of Introduction of Allergenic Foods in Breast-Fed Infants," *New England Journal of Medicine*, 2016 May, 5:374(18):1733-43.

Perkin, M., et al., "Enquiring About Tolerance (EAT) Study: Feasibility of an Early Allergenic Food Introduction Regimen," *Journal of Allergy and Clinical Immunology*, 2016 May; 137(5): 1477–1486.e8.

Tran, MM, et al., "The Effects of Feeding Practices On Food Sensitization In A Canadian Birth Cohort," *American Journal of Respiratory and Critical Care Medicine*, 193;2016:A6694, May 2018.

Meeting of The American Thoracic Society, "Early Introduction of Allergenic Foods Reduces Risk of Food Sensitization," May 18, 2016.

"Infant Feeding and Allergy Prevention," *Australasian Society of Clinical Immunology and Allergy*, May 2016, www.allergy.org.au.

"Addendum Guidelines for the Prevention of Peanut Allergy in the United States," National Institute of Allergy and Infectious Disease, January 2017, niaid.nih.gov.

Hoffman, B. et al, "What Pediatricians Are Advising on Infant Peanut Introduction," *Annals of Allergy, Asthma, and Immunology*, November 2017, Volume 119, Issue 5.

Chapter VI

Coon, E., MD, et al., "Update on Pediatric Overuse," *Pediatrics*, Volume 139, number 2, February 2017.

Carroll, A., MD, "It's Hard for Doctors to Unlearn Things. That's Costly for All of Us," *New York Times*, September 10, 2018.

Lohr, K., "Rating the Strength of Scientific Evidence: Relevance for Quality Improvement Programs," *International Journal for Quality in Health Care*, 2004 Feb;16(1):9-18.

Saarni, S., "Evidence Based Medicine Guidelines: A Solution to Rationing or Politics Disguised as Science," *Journal of Medical Ethics*, 2004 Apr;30(2):171-5.

Feeney, M., et al., "Impact of Peanut Consumption in the LEAP Study: Feasibility, Growth, and Nutrition," *Journal of Allergy and Clinical Immunology*, Volume 138, Number 4, 2016 Oct;138(4):1108-1118.

Perkin, M., et al., "Enquiring About Tolerance (EAT) Study: Feasibility of an Early Allergenic Food Introduction Regimen," *Journal of Allergy and Clinical Immunology*, 2016 May; 137(5): 1477–1486.e8.

Anderson, J., "Confused About Introducing Solids?," Australian Breastfeeding Association.

Wilson, C., "Should Babies Be Given Solids Earlier to Prevent Food Allergies?," *New Scientist*, 10/19/2015.

Abrams, E., "Early Solid Food Introduction: Role in Food Allergy Prevention and Implications for Breastfeeding," *The Journal of Pediatrics*, May 2017, Volume 184, pages 13-18.

Bock, S., MD, et al., "Fatalities Due to Anaphylactic Reactions to Foods," *J Allergy and Clinical Immunology*, 2001;107;191-3.

Rudders, S., MD, et al., "Age-related Differences in the Clinical Presentation of Food-induced Anaphylaxis," *Journal of Pediatrics*, 2011 Feb: 158(2):326-328.

Topal, E., et al., "Anaphylaxis in Infancy Compared with Older Children," *Allergy and Asthma Proceedings*, May-June 2013, 34(3):233-8.

Sicherer, S., "UpToDate," Nov 29,2017. (Original reference: Grabenhenrich, LB, et al., "Anaphylaxis in Children and Adolescents: The European Anaphylaxis Registry," *Journal of Allergy and Clinical Immunology*, 2016;137(4):1128. Epub 2016 Jan 21.)

Turner, P. MD, et, al., "Implementing Primary Prevention for Peanut Allergy at a Population Level," *Journal of the American Medical Association*, 2017 March 21;317(11):1111-1112.

Koplin, J., et al., "Understanding the Feasibility and Implications of Implementing Early Peanut Introduction For Prevention of Peanut Allergy," *The Journal of Allergy and Clinical Immunology*, Oct. 2016, Volume 138, Issue 4, Pages 1131–1141.e2.

Hallemann, C., "New Childhood Allergy Guidelines Recommend Early Exposure to Eggs, Peanuts," *Parenting Magazine* online.

Fleischer, D., "New Recommendations for Preventing Food Allergies," *Contemporary Pediatrics* October 25, 2016.

Young, M., MD, "The Peanut Allergy Answer Book," Third Edition, 2013.

Abrams, E., MD, et al., "Timing of Introduction of Allergenic Solids for Infants at High Risk," Canadian Pediatric Society, January 24, 2019.

Koplin, J., et al, "The HealthNuts Study," *International Journal of Epidemiology*, Volume 44, Issue 4, 1 August 2015, pages 1161–1171.

Tikkanen, E., "Associations of Fitness, Physical Activity, Strength, and Genetic Risk With Cardiovascular Disease: Longitudinal Analyses in the U.K. Biobank Study," *Circulation*, 2018 June 12;137(24):2583-2591.

"Physical Activity Helps Fight Genetic Risk of Heart Disease," Stanford Medicine News Center, med.stanford.edu.

Bilaver, L., PhD, "Socioeconomic Disparities in the Economic Impact of Childhood Food Allergy," *Pediatrics*, Volume 137, Number 5, May 2016.

Turner, P., MD, "Fatal Anaphylaxis: Mortality Rate and Risk Factors," *Journal of Allergy and Clinical Immunology Practice*, 2017 Sep-Oct; 5(5): 1169–1178.

Altmann, T., MD, "What to Feed Your Baby," HarperOne, 2016.

Greene, A., MD, "2011 White Paper:Why White Rice Cereal for Babies Must Go," online, Dr.Greene.com.

Cha, A., "Americans Junk Food Habits Start in Toddler Years," *The Washington Post*, April 6, 2016.

"US Infants' Sugar Consumption Exceeds Adult Recommendations," Meeting News from the American Society for Nutrition Scientific Sessions and Annual Meeting, June 11, 2018.

Birch, L., MD, et al., "Influences on the Development of Children's Eating Behaviours: From Infancy to Adolescence," *Canadian Journal of Dietetic Practice and Research*, 2007; 68(1): s1–s56.

"Nutrition for Healthy Term Infants: Recommendations from Six to 24 Months," A Joint Statement of Health Canada, Canadian Paediatric Society, Dietitians of Canada, and Breastfeeding Committee for Canada.

Jiwa, M., "Doctors and Medical Science," *Australasian Medical Journal*, September 9, 2012; 5(8): 462-467.

Allen, K., Professor at Murdoch Children's Research Institute, Department of Allergy and Immunology, University of Melbourne, Results from the LEAP study.

Chapter VII

Gupta, R., et al., Research Presented at the American College of Asthma, Allergy, and Immunology Annual Scientific Meeting, October 2017, Boston, MA.

Silverberg, J., et al., "Associations of Childhood Eczema Severity: a US Population-based Study," *Dermatitis*, 2014 May-June;25(3):107-14.

"Egg Allergy Overview," American College of Asthma, Allergy and Immunology website.

Du Toit, G., et al., "Randomized Trial of Peanut Consumption in Infants At Risk for Peanut Allergy," *New England Journal of Medicine*, February 23, 2015; 372:803-813.

"Eczema May Play a Key Role in the Development of Food Allergy in Infants, Study Suggests," *Science News*, July 19, 2013; King's College London.

Chapter VIII

"Meningococcal Disease," Centers for Disease Control and Prevention, cdc.gov.

"Statistics and Disease Facts," National Meningitis Association, nmaus.org.

Harrison, L., "Epidemiological Profile of Meningococcal Disease in the United States," *Clinical Infectious Diseases*, Volume 50, Issue Supplement 2, March 1, 2010, pages S37–S44.

Shepard, CW, et al., "Cost-effectiveness of Conjugate Meningococcal Vaccination Strategies in the United States," *Pediatrics*, 2005 May;115(5):1220-32.

"Common Knee Operation in Elderly Constitutes Low Value Care, New Study Concludes," Johns Hopkins Medicine, February 28, 2018.

Englund, M., "Meniscectomy and Osteoarthritis: What is the Cause and What is the Effect?," *Future Rheumatology,* (2006) **1**(2), 207–215.

"The Evolution of Meniscal Surgery: From Impunity to Importance," *Orthopedics Today,* July 2005.

Shivonen, R., MD, et al., "Arthroscopic Partial Meniscectomy versus Sham Surgery for a Degenerative Meniscal Tear," *New England Journal of Medicine,* December 26, 2013; 369:2515-2524.

Marsh, J., et al., "Cost-effectiveness Analysis of Arthroscopic Surgery Compared with Non-operative Management for Osteoarthritis of the Knee," *British Medical Journal Open,* January 12, 2016, Volume 6, Issue 1.

Mullaney, T., "The Most Common Knee Surgery for Seniors is Costly, and Usually a Waste," cnbc.com, April 6, 2018.

Jain, S., et al., "Community-Acquired Pneumonia Requiring Hospitalization among U.S. Children," *New England Journal of Medicine,* February 26, 2015; 372:835-845.

Sifferlin, A., "13% of Americans Take Antidepressants," *Time Magazine,* August 15, 2017.

Khan, A., "Antidepressants versus Placebo in Major Depression: An Overview," *World Psychiatry,* 2015 Oct; 14(3): 294–300.

O'Hara, M., et al., "Why 'Big Pharma' Stopped Searching for the Next Prozac," *The Guardian,* January 27, 2016.

"Group A Strep (GAS) Disease," Surveillance, Centers for Disease Control and Prevention, cdc.gov.

Worrall, G., "Acute Sore Throat," *Canadian Family Physician,* 2011 Jul; 57(7): 791–794.

Wolford, R., "Pediatric Pharyngitis," Clerkship Directors in Emergency Medicine, cdemcurriculum.com.

McMurray, K., "Taking Chances with Strep Throat," *Hospital Pediatrics,* 2015 Oct;5(10):552-554.

World Heart Federation, "Treating Sore Throat Should Be Part of Strategy to Prevent Rheumatic Heart Disease," *Science Daily,* September 26, 2013, sciencedaily.com.

Pfoh, E., "Burden and Economic Cost of Group A Streptococcal Pharyngitis," *Pediatrics,* 2008 Feb;121(2): 229-34.

Newman, D., "Antibiotics for Strep Do More Harm Than Good," *Emergency Physicians Monthly,* epmonthly.com.

Kothari, S., "Of History, Half-truths, and Rheumatic Fever," *Annals of Pediatric Cardiology,* 2013 July-Dec: 6(2): 117-120.

Hajar, R., "Rheumatic Fever and Rheumatic Heart Disease a Historical Perspective," *Heart Views,* 2016 July-September; 17(3): 120-126.

Hayes, C., "The Secret Reason We Treat Strep Throat," chadhayesmd.com.

Gordis, L., "The Virtual Disappearance of Rheumatic Fever in the United States: Lessons in the Rise and Fall of Disease, T. Duckett Jones Memorial Lecture," *Circulation,* 1985 December; 72(6): 1155-62.

"Rheumatic Fever," Mayo Clinic, mayoclinic.org.

Patterson, K., "What Doctors Don't Know (Almost Everything)," *New York Times,* May 5, 2002.

Lohr, K., "Rating the Strength of Scientific Evidence: Relevance for Quality Improvement Programs," *International Journal for Quality in Health Care,* 2004 February;16(1):9-18.

"Total Number of Registered Clinical Studies Worldwide Since 2000," *Statista,* statista.com.

Society for Clinical Trials, LEAP Selected as the 2015 David Sackett Trial of the Year, sctweb.org.

Chapter IX

Wahl, B., "Burden of Streptococcus pneumoniae and Haemophilus influenza type b Disease in Children in the Era of Conjugate Vaccines: Global, Regional, and National Estimates for 2000–15," *Lancet Global Health*, Volume 6, Issue 7, PE744-E757, July 01, 2018.

"Simply Peanut™ Launches Peanut Introduction Product for Infants Four Months Plus," *Digital Journal*, February 20, 2017.

"Launch of Hello, Peanut! Marks First and Only Product Available for Parents to Safely Introduce Peanuts to Infants," *PR Newswire*, March 7, 2016.

Antera Therapeutics Announces First and Only Commercial Product Based on LEAP for Early Peanut Introduction, March 5, 2016, PRNewswire.

Zweig, D., "Shell Shock: Why is a Startup Charging Parents $180 for $2 Worth of Peanut Butter?," *The Verge*, August 4, 2016.

SpoonfulOne website, spoonfulone.com

Raphael, R., "Can A Spoonful Of This Powder Help Prevent Children's Food Allergies?," *Fast Company*, October 19, 2017.

Chapter X

Lack, G., et al., "Factors Associated with the Development of Peanut

Allergy in Childhood," *New England Journal of Medicine*, March 13, 2003; 348:977-985

Brough, HA, et al., "Peanut Protein in Household Dust is Related to Household Peanut Consumption and is Biologically Active," *Journal of Allergy and Clinical Immunology*, 2013 Sep;132(3):630-638.

"Eczema May Play Key Role in Development of Food Allergy in Infants," Kings College London, July 18, 2013.

Chapter XI

Fleischer, D., "The Impact of Breastfeeding on the Development of Allergic Disease," UpToDate.com.

Pitt, T., MD, et al., "Reduced Risk of Peanut Sensitization Following Exposure Through Breast-feeding and Early Peanut Introduction," *Journal of Allergy and Clinical Immunology*, 2018 February;141(2):620-625.e1.

Koplin, J., PhD, et al., "Understanding the Feasibility and Implications of Implementing Early Peanut Introduction for Prevention of Peanut Allergy," *The Journal of Allergy and Clinical Immunology*, 2016 October;138(4):1131-1141.e2.

Turner, PJ, et al., "Implementing Primary Prevention for Peanut Allergy at a Population Level," *Journal of the American Medical Association*, 2017 March 21;317(11):1111-1112.

Stukus, D., MD, VIDEO: "New Early Peanut Introduction Guidelines Must Undo 'Years of Misconceptions'," Highlights from American College of Allergy, Asthma, and Immunology, Oct, 28, 2017, healio.com.

Perkin, M., et al., "Enquiring About Tolerance (EAT) study: Feasibility of an Early Allergenic Food Introduction Regimen," *Journal of Allergy and Clinical Immunology,* 2016 May; 137(5): 1477–1486.e8.

Perkin, M., et al., "Randomized Trial of Introduction of Allergenic Foods in Breast-Fed Infants," *New England Journal of Medicine,* 2016 May 5;374(18):1733-43.

Du Toit, G., et al., "Effect of Avoidance on Peanut Allergy after Early Peanut Consumption," *New England Journal of Medicine,* 2016; 374:1435-1443, April 14, 2016.

"LEAP-ON Study Results," Immune Tolerance Network, leapstudy.co.uk

Matti, M., LEAP Co-Author: "How Not to Stress Out About Early Peanut Introduction," *Allergic Living Magazine,* January 12, 2017.

Wood, R., "Understanding and Managing Sesame Allergy," Food Allergy Research & Education, foodallergy.org, October 14, 2015.

"Efforts Continue to Add Sesame As Top Allergen," Food Allergy Research & Education, foodallergy.org, May 8, 2016.

Smith, G., "A LEAP into an Allergic Culture Change," *Allergic Living*, March 15, 2016.

Frazier, A., MD, ScM, et al., "Prospective Study of Peripregnancy Consumption of Peanuts or Tree Nuts by Mothers and the Risk of Peanut or Tree Nut Allergy in Their Offspring," *Journal of the American Medical Association Pediatrics,* 2014;168(2):156-162.

About the Author

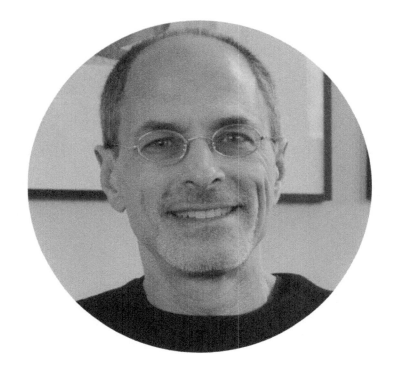

DR. RON SUNOG GREW UP in New York, earned his MD at Boston University's accelerated six-year medical program, and completed his Residency and Chief Residency in Pediatrics at Boston City Hospital. He lives near Boston with his family and has been taking care of infants and children of all ages in pediatric practice for over thirty years. Having long had a special interest in nutrition, he was inspired by the LEAP study to create Eat The Eight to inform parents about infant feeding to reduce the risk of developing food allergy. In 2017, he joined Puffworks as Medical Advisor to help create Puffworks baby, a better way to introduce peanut to infants to help reduce the risk of developing peanut allergy.

About *The Nasiona*

Birds then came, bringing in **seeds**, *and our pile became an oasis of life.*

Pojawiły się ptaki, przynosząc **nasiona** *i nasza skądinąd jałowa górka stała się oazą życia. (Polish)*

The Nasiona is a community of creatives whose mission is to cultivate the seeds of nonfiction. We do this through a nonfiction literary magazine, podcast, and publishing house, as well as by offering editing services, literary contests, and an internship program.

In an age when telling the difference between reality and delusion is frighteningly labyrinthine, we focus on creative works based on facts, truth-seeking, human concerns, real events, and real people, with a personal touch.

From liminal lives to the marginalized, and everything in between, we glimpse into different, at times extraordinary, worlds to promote narrative-led nonfiction stories and art that explore the spectrum of human experience. We believe that the subjective can offer its own reality and reveal truths some facts can't discover.

We're a diversity-friendly organization that values multicultural and multi-experience perspectives on what it means to be human. We look to erase borders, tackle taboos, resist conventions, explore the known and unknown, and rename ourselves to claim ourselves.

We feature creative nonfiction and nonfiction poetry, a column on memoir writing, visual art, and interview interesting individuals from all over.

We publish continuously, on a rolling basis, and accept submissions from emerging and established authors and content creators.

Our Podcast brings the magazine to life.

We offer editing services for poetry, fiction, and nonfiction manuscripts of any length.

Our publishing house will begin publishing nonfiction book-length manuscripts in 2019.

Our internship program aims to contribute to the development of editors, journalists, writers, scholars, and those interested in the publishing industry.

With our literary contests, we look to identify and celebrate some of the best original, unpublished creative nonfiction and nonfiction poetry out there.

We founded *The Nasiona* in the summer of 2018 in California. Though based in hilly San Francisco, the world is our home. Help us cultivate this pile of seeds and we'll do our best to create a worthy oasis for human life to not only exist but flourish.

The Nasiona depends on voluntary contributions from readers like you. We hope the value of our work to the community is worth your patronage. If you like what we do, please show this by financially supporting our work through our Patreon platform.

https://www.patreon.com/join/TheNasiona

Please follow *The Nasiona* on Twitter, Instagram, and Facebook for regular updates: @TheNasiona

nasiona.mail@gmail.com

https://thenasiona.com/

Made in the USA
Middletown, DE
27 September 2020